AN A-Z FAMILY GUIDE

NATURAL
· HEALTH
· REMEDIES

AN A-Z FAMILY GUIDE

NATURAL · HEALTH · REMEDIES

JANET MACCARO, PH.D., C.N.C.

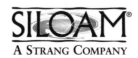

A STRANG COMPANY

NATURAL HEALTH REMEDIES by Janet Maccaro, Ph.D.
Published by Siloam
A Strang Company
600 Rinehart Road
Lake Mary, Florida 32746
www.siloam.com

Scripture quotations marked KJV are from the King James Version of the Bible.

Scripture quotations marked NAS are from the New American Standard Bible. Copyright © 1960, 1962, 1963, 1968, 1971, 1972, 1973, 1975, 1977 by the Lockman Foundation. Used by permission. (www.Lockman.org)

Scripture quotations marked NIV are from the Holy Bible, New International Version. Copyright © 1973, 1978, 1984, International Bible Society. Used by permission.

Scripture quotations marked NKJV are from the New King James Version of the Bible. Copyright © 1979, 1980, 1982 by Thomas Nelson, Inc., publishers. Used by permission.

Cover design by Judith McKittrick
Interior design by David Bilby

This book is not intended to provide medical advice or to take the place of medical advice and treatment from your personal physician. Readers are advised to consult their own doctors or other qualified health professionals regarding the treatment of their medical problems. Neither the publisher nor the author takes any responsibility for any possible consequences from any treatment, action or application of medicine, supplement, herb or preparation to any person reading or following the information in this book. If readers are taking prescription medications, they should consult with their physicians and not take themselves off of medicines to start supplementation without the proper supervision of a physician.

Library of Congress Cataloging-in-Publication Data

Maccaro, Janet C.
   Natural health remedies / Janet Maccaro.
      p. cm.
   Includes bibliographical references.
Summary: This book offers an A to Z guide explaining physical, emotional and spiritual root causes of many common diseases and ailments. It also provides alternative, natural solutions from vitamins, minerals, herbs and food supplements.
   ISBN 0-88419-930-4 (pbk. : alk. paper)
   1. Naturopathy. 2. Dietary supplements. I. Title.
RZ440 .M33 2003
615.5'35—dc21
                        2002152107
            05 06 07 08 — 12 11 10 9 8
         Printed in the United States of America

AUTHOR'S NOTE: While we present here some valuable and helpful protocols and therapies that come from cultures that are not based in a Christian world-view, we in no way want to be perceived as promoting other religions or non-Christian philosophies. We simply have extracted therapeutic protocols that can be helpful in promoting health, understanding that our spiritual well-being depends on our personal relationship with Christ.

—JANET MACCARO, PH.D., C.N.C.

Because modern medicine was not available in biblical times, treating a sick person in that culture involved making them as comfortable as possible and praying to God for healing. While it is true that in today's world of medical science we can do for patients much more than our forefathers could in terms of medical intervention, every good doctor knows the powerful role that faith and prayer still play in modern-day medical miracles.

Even physicians who do not personally believe in the power of faith and prayer have to admit that people of faith often experience swifter healing and sustain longer-term recoveries than those without a confession of faith. And they have a definite advantage when facing hopeless conditions that demand miraculous turnarounds.

Realizing that we can never achieve enough experience and education to live independently from faith in God, I dedicate this book to His promise:

> "I will restore health to you and heal you of your wounds," says the Lord.
>
> —Jeremiah 30:17, NKJV

May this book be an extension of His healing grace.

CONTENTS

LIST OF CHARTS

HEALTH UPDATES

INTRODUCTION

You are about to embark on an incredible journey into natural health. This is a journey I have taken personally. My passion or burning desire to write this family guide to natural health is birthed out of twenty years of my own health struggles in which I tried to find answers to the myriad of physical symptoms that I endured. I want to offer you the profound secrets of my journey to health, hope and healing in a natural, drugless format that addresses body balance and gives plentiful encouragement.

TAKING THE CHALLENGE

If you are seeking to take more responsibility for your state of health and well-being, this book is written just for you. God designed our bodies with a healing system that can handle most health problems without outside intervention. In this era of knowledge explosion, many people are searching for better answers for their health needs and those of their families.

You will find the format of this health guide to be "user friendly," which will encourage you to "get back on track" in terms of your health. You can use this reference book as your family "self-care manual." Refer to it often. Become an educated, active participant in the building and maintenance of vibrant health.

A CHRISTIAN PERSPECTIVE

This book, written from a Christian perspective to bring healing to your body, mind and spirit, is dramatically different from other natural health reference books, which may be steeped in New Age beliefs, Eastern mysticism and the occult. The Bible clearly outlines good dietary principles that have been proven time and time again to be health building. Because the Bible teaches that our bodies are the temples of the Holy Spirit, Christians believe that we must take care of our "temples." (See 1 Corinthians 6:19.) The world of natural medicine can be of tremendous benefit in this regard. Herbs, minerals, vitamins and other modalities can help to balance, cleanse and nurture our bodies to prevent disease.

Christians look to God as the source of all healing. They also believe that He has supplied every "herb of the field" as support for the health of our bodies. And Christians realize that total health depends not only on the state of the body, but also the mind and spirit as well. To neglect one of these areas means that the health needs of one-third of our being are not addressed. Vibrant health is not possible unless the "total person" is regenerated.

The New Age belief system focuses on the "self" as the healer. It teaches that a person can achieve "self-realization" that will open the door to spiritual realms where other "beings" serve as teachers to aid in attaining mastery of the self. Christians do not attempt "self" mastery; we have a Master, Jesus Christ. We look to His promises for our health: "'I will restore health to you and heal you of your wounds,' says the LORD" (Jer. 30:17, NKJV). And we follow His design for our health.

As you read this family guide to natural medicine, you will learn much about your body and its grand design. You will be armed against the attacks that come against it—body, mind and spirit. You will learn to take advantage of His gifts to us: herbs, vitamins, minerals and more. We can use them to build, strengthen and heal our bodies.

Take advantage of what God has provided. Partake of all of the good things in nature that He has sent to us bathed in sunshine, washed by the rain, sown by the wind and nurtured by His hand. And learn to enjoy the favor of God on your life as you determine to...

Glorify God in your body and in your spirit, which are God's.
—1 CORINTHIANS 6:20, NKJV

Part One

Natural Medicine 101

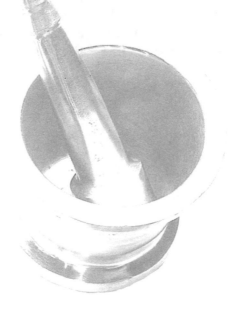

PART ONE

———◆·▸◆·◆———

NATURAL MEDICINE 101

Yet his [man's] days shall be one hundred and twenty years.
—GENESIS 6:3, NKJV

Our life expectancy can be extended by ten to forty extra years! A breakthrough has occurred between traditional medicine and alternative healthcare. Once at opposite ends of the spectrum, these two schools of medical treatment have come together, working in an unprecedented way to heal the total person—body, mind and spirit!

I have experienced both ends of the healing spectrum personally, which birthed my passion for helping persons overcome physical illness, emotional pain and spiritual depletion. This family guide will serve your family for years to come, arming you with the information to prevent illness, heal and strengthen the body and feed the soul. It is my prayer that this book will replace fear with fact, hopelessness with healing and despair with renewal!

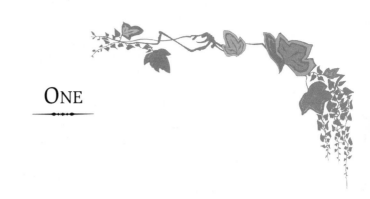

ONE

NATURAL MEDICINE 101

My son, attend to my words; incline thine ear unto my sayings...For they are life unto those that find them, and health to all their flesh.

—PROVERBS 4:20, 22, KJV

It is the premise of natural medicine that the body has a God-given, built-in ability to heal itself and that the role of the physician is to aid or enhance this process with natural therapies such as dietary changes, herbs, vitamins and minerals. Natural medicine is noninvasive. It supports the body by feeding, balancing and cleansing all the channels of elimination.

Proponents of natural medicine view the person as a whole being—body, mind and spirit. Your emotional and mental state, in addition to your physical health, must be addressed and understood when seeking to understand factors that cause a particular health challenge.

GETTING TO THE ROOT OF IT!

Natural medicine does not simply seek to suppress symptoms with drugs and so forth, but it attempts to discover and eliminate the root cause of disease. It examines the body, observing its five main systems: the digestive, respiratory, endocrine, circulatory and immune systems. And it looks at the four major elimination channels: the bowels, skin, lungs and kidneys. Natural medicine does so in order to determine treatment.

Natural medicine educates patients by involving them in their healthcare. They become active participants in their personal well-being. They learn to be more accountable for their dietary lifestyles. And they understand that, because illness can be the result of spiritual or emotional unrest, a strong prayer life is a very wise medicine to include in the healing process.

Focus on prevention

Finally, natural medicine teaches not only the *treatment* of disease but also its *prevention* by instilling dietary and lifestyle habits that promote health. Why wait for disease to strike before you begin to focus on your health? It is hard to play "catch up" when it comes to your health. While it is true that God wonderfully designed our bodies' healing systems with remarkable recuperative ability, prevention is far and away the best way to go.

We step back in awe as we learn what natural medicine teaches us about the wonder of our bodies and how they are equipped to fight disease. We marvel at God's workmanship when we stop, look and listen to what the body is saying through disease symptoms in order to inform us when we are doing something wrong.

It is still a sad fact that many medical schools do not teach disease prevention as a part of healthcare. This book will educate you in a way that will give you more control over your health problems. Armed with that knowledge, you will become an important part of the decision-making process regarding your health.

Every health-building recommendation in this book has been thoroughly researched and used clinically by thousands of nutritionists and physicians. Some of them I discovered and used personally in my quest for wellness that spanned over twenty years. I invite you to use them all to add years to your life and life to your years!

The World of Vitamins

Experts agree that one of the best ways to safeguard your health is to eat only the healthiest foods you can find. Plenty of fresh fruits, vegetables and whole grains along with low-fat dairy are the general recommendation. This is because of all of the "phytochemicals" or vitamins, minerals and fiber that are naturally occurring and health protective.

But knowing that we all are under more stress these days from work, family and the pressures of life in general, most experts now agree that a multivitamin/mineral supplement makes perfect sense. A good vitamin supplement can close nutritional gaps left by poor dietary habits. Evidence suggests that vitamins may increase our "health span," which means active years that are free from chronic illness.

Your need for nutritional supplements

The outdated theory of mainstream medicine that holds that you can get all of the vitamins and minerals you need from your diet is slowly dying out. More and more physicians realize that, while it may have been true that our grandparents received all the nutrition they required from their foods, this is simply not the case in our generation. Mineral-depleted soils and chemical agribusiness farming and marketing methods almost guarantee that you will not get anywhere near the ideal nutritional value that you need for health from the foods you buy at the supermarket.

You may have heard this statement: "Taking vitamins results only in expensive urine." It is true that all substances are eventually excreted, but what vitamins do on their way through your blood stream is health building and life enhancing. Keeping your body blanketed with the full spectrum of vitamins and minerals is like an insurance policy, which will help to guard you against physical decline and degenerative disease.

HOW VITAMINS WORK TO STRENGTHEN AND SUPPORT YOUR BODY

The following chart provides the main benefits of each vitamin and the most common food sources in which they are found. I have listed the B vitamins separately, even though they work together as a team to maintain health. It is helpful to eat more foods that have vitamins your health condition needs to heal. However, as we mentioned, it is necessary to take supplements of those vitamins to be sure to get adequate amounts the body needs.

VITAMIN BENEFITS AND SOURCES		
VITAMIN	**BENEFITS**	**FOOD SOURCES**
Vitamin A (retinol)	Maintains healthy vision; assists with formation and growth of epithelial tissue (membranes lining eye and mouth cavities, stomach and intestines, lungs and other organs); assists growth and reproduction; assists immune system; protects against cancer.	green and yellow fruits and vegetables; fish liver oils; herbs such as alfalfa, paprika, parsley, red clover and many others
Vitamin C	Builds collagen; maintains healthy gum, teeth and blood vessels.	grapefruit, oranges, strawberries, spinach, cabbage, melons, tomatoes
Vitamin D	Aids in calcium absorption; assists with growth of bones and teeth	salmon, tuna, eggs, milk, butter Other sources: sunlight
Vitamin E	Protects cells from damage; improves circulation; is an antioxidant; necessary for tissue repair; important in cancer prevention	apples, peanuts, spinach, blackberries, wheat germ, nut and vegetable oils, mangos

VITAMIN	BENEFITS	FOOD SOURCES
Vitamin K	Provides blood clotting	eggs, carrots, avocados, tomatoes, parsley, cabbage, spinach, broccoli, Brussels sprouts
Vitamin B₁ (thiamine)	Enhances circulation; is an antioxidant; assists in production of hydrochloric acid; assists in blood formation; energizes; promotes growth and learning capacity	egg yolks, fish, wheat germ, oatmeal, peanuts, poultry
Vitamin B₂ (riboflavin)	Helps in formation of red blood cells	cheese, milk, egg yolks, spinach, mushrooms, broccoli
Vitamin B₃ (niacin, niacinamide, nicotinic acid)	Provides healthy skin and good circulation	carrots, wheat germ, brewer's yeast, cheese, peanuts, milk
Vitamin B₅ (pantothenic acid)	Is an antistress vitamin; plays a role in the production of abnormal hormones	eggs, royal jelly, brewer's yeast, liver, mushrooms
Vitamin B₆ (pyridoxine)	Promotes cancer immunity; prevents arteriosclerosis by inhibiting homocysteine	brewer's yeast, walnuts, eggs, spinach, peas, chicken, bananas
Vitamin B₁₂ (cyanocobalamin)	Prevents anemia; helps utilization of iron	seafood, dairy, eggs, brewer's yeast, milk
Biotin	Aids in metabolism of carbohydrates, fats and proteins; aids in fatty acid production; promotes healthy skin and nails	soybeans, whole grains, brewer's yeast, meat, milk, poultry, cooked egg yolks
Coenzyme Q₁₀ (ubiquinone)	Is a powerful antioxidant; is important for the production of energy in every cell of the body	salmon, sardines, mackerel, peanuts, spinach, beef
Folic acid	Aids energy production; aids formation of red blood cells	chicken, tuna, milk, liver, brown rice, salmon, wheat germ, dates

VITAMIN	BENEFITS	FOOD SOURCES
Choline	Helps disorders of the nervous system; is necessary for proper transmission of nerve impulses from the brain through the central nervous system. Without it brain function and memory are impaired.	soybean, egg yolks, meat, lecithin
Inositol	Has a calming effect; reduces cholesterol levels; helps remove fats from the liver; essential for hair growth	lecithin, meats, raisins, whole grains, milk, brewer's yeast
Beta carotene	Is a vitamin A precursor (converts to vitamin A in the liver); is a power free-radical scavenger (antioxidant); strengthens immune response; helps guard against stroke and heart disease; helps with tissue repair, healthy skin and mucous membranes	carrots, yams, squash, spinach, broccoli
PABA	Is an antioxidant; protects against skin cancer; may help restore gray hair to original color if the condition is stress related	liver, spinach, mushrooms, molasses

Health Update — The Value of Nutritional Supplements

The more I learn about nutritional supplements, the more I discover nutritional components that can help nearly everyone. In fact, I consider prescribing and individualizing of programs of vita-nutrients to be one of the two pillars of nutritional medicine.[1]

—DR. ROBERT ATKINS

Choosing a Multivitamin

When choosing a multivitamin, it is important to remember that not all vitamins are created equal. Here are some considerations for helping you to make the best choices:

- Look for the "USP" number on the label. This number gives you the percentage of the product that has been formulated to dissolve after one hour in body fluids. The percentage should be as high as possible and will vary from product to product.

- Make sure the iron in your multivitamin is either ferrous fumarate or ferrous sulfate because they are the most absorbable forms.

- For best absorption, take your multivitamin with meals and not on an empty stomach. Otherwise you may experience nausea.

- Another important tip is to make sure that you take your multivitamin with a meal that contains a little fat. The fat-soluble vitamins (A, D and E) need a little fat to get inside your system and go to work.

Adding Essential Minerals

A good multivitamin also contains essential minerals the body needs for optimum health. Vitamins and minerals work together in synergy to boost and support our body's systems. Every living cell depends on minerals for proper function and structure. The balance of your body depends upon proper levels and ratios of different minerals. Minerals are crucial for proper nerve function, regulation of muscle tone, formation of blood and bone and composition of body fluids. The entire cardiovascular system relies heavily on proper mineral balance.

The following chart provides the main benefits of each mineral and the most common food sources where the minerals are found. Even though we can get the minerals from some food sources, it is sometimes necessary to supplement with these minerals in order to get sufficient amounts for our bodies' needs.

MINERAL BENEFITS AND SOURCES

MINERAL	BENEFITS	FOOD SOURCES
Calcium	Provides strong bones, teeth, muscle and nerve function; aids in blood clotting	salmon, sardines, yogurt, milk, cheese, broccoli, green beans, almonds, turnip greens
Chloride	Aids digestion; works with sodium to maintain fluid balance	salted foods
Chromium	Provides proper carbohydrate metabolism	broccoli, orange and grapefruit juice, brown sugar, cheese, brewer's yeast
Copper	Aids in formation of blood cells and connective tissues	oysters, shellfish, cocoa, cherries, mushrooms, gelatin, eggs, fish, legumes
Fluoride	Strengthens tooth enamel	fish, tea, fluoridated water
Iodine	Maintains proper thyroid function	iodized salt, shrimp, lobster, oysters, spinach, milk
Manganese	Aids calcium, phosphorous and magnesium metabolism; provides essential support for healthy bones	avocados, seeds, nuts, egg yolks, blueberries, pineapples, legumes
Boron	Needed in trace amounts for proper calcium absorption (elderly need 2 or 3 mg daily)	grapes, grains, apples, carrots, leafy vegetables
Zinc	Sharpens taste and smell; is essential for prostate gland function and proper reproductive organ growth; may help curb acne by aiding in the regulation of oil glands; is wonderful for the immune system; aids in wound healing; is required for proper collagen formation and protein synthesis; protects the liver from chemical assaults; is essential for proper bone formation	mushrooms, egg yolks, sardines, whole grains, pumpkinseeds, sunflower seeds, liver

MINERAL	BENEFITS	FOOD SOURCES
Phosphorous	Is important for tooth and bone formation, kidney function, cell growth and contraction of the heart muscle	pumpkinseeds, sunflower seeds, dairy products, eggs, fish, dried fruit, nuts, salmon, poultry, corn, whole grains, sodas/soft drinks
Iron	Needed for the production and oxygenation of red blood cells; is essential for healthy immune system	liver, meats, poultry, eggs, fish, almonds, avocados, black strap molasses, brewer's yeast, prunes, pumpkins, raisins, beets, peaches, pears
Germanium	Carries oxygen to the cells, which in turn boosts immunity	mushrooms, garlic, onions
Magnesium	Necessary to prevent the calcification of soft tissue; helps prevent muscle tightness, dizziness, PMS and high blood pressure; aids in formation of bone	dairy, meats, fish, nuts, molasses, brewer's yeast, avocados, bananas
Molybdenum	Promotes normal cell function	dark leafy greens, peas, beans, cereal
Potassium	Helps maintain regular heart rhythm; is important for nervous system function	bananas, apricots, fish, dairy, garlic, nuts, yams, wheat bran
Selenium	Inhibits the oxidation of blood fats (lipids); protects the immune system from free-radical damage	brown rice, salmon, broccoli, brewer's yeast, dairy products, garlic, liver
Sulfur	Disinfects the blood; protects against radiation; needed for the synthesis of collagen; is essential as a skin nutrient	garlic, wheat germ, onions, soybeans, eggs, fish, Brussels sprouts

I suggest you use the following Daily RDA Chart for Vitamins and Minerals to choose your multivitamin and mineral supplements.[2]

DAILY RDA CHART FOR VITAMINS AND MINERALS			
VITAMINS	**DOSAGE**	**MINERALS**	**DOSAGE**
Vitamin A	10,000 IU	Calcium	1,500 mg
Beta carotene	15,000 IU	Chromium (GTF)	200 mcg
Vitamin B_1	50 mg	Copper	3 mg
Vitamin B_2	50 mg	Iodine	225 mcg
Vitamin B_3 (niacin)	100 mg	Iron (only if a deficiency exists)	18 mg
Vitamin B_5 (pantothenic acid)	100 mg	Magnesium	750–1,000 mg
		Manganese	10 mg
Vitamin B_6	50 mg	Molybdenum	30 mg
Vitamin B_{12}	300 mcg	Potassium	99 mg
Biotin	300 mcg	Selenium	200 mcg
Choline	100 mg	Zinc	50 mg
Folic acid	800 mcg		
Inositol	100 mcg		
PABA	50 mg		
Vitamin C (ester and ascorbic)	500 mg		
Vitamin D	400 IU		
Vitamin E	600 IU		
Vitamin K	100 mcg		

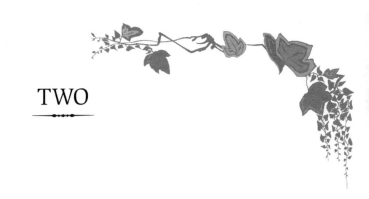

TWO

HEALING HERBS—A TO Z

Herbal plants are time-tested and approved sources of healing that are truly gifts from God. He has given us every herb of the field for the healing and strengthening of our bodies. (See Psalm 104:14.) Did you know that many of our modern-day medicines are derived from herbs? Researchers all over the world know that herbs are very powerful and effective resources for healing.

Research is ongoing to discover how and why herbs can bring balance and healing to our lives. In Europe, herbs have been used as medicines for centuries and continue to be used on a daily basis. Europeans have confidence in herbal therapy. Now thousands of Americans are embracing herbs as a way to prevent or treat illness.

As we explore these wonderful healing plants, let me stress that they can have powerful effects on our bodies and must be treated with respect. Proper education in their healing properties as well as cautions for their use are key to securing their potential benefits for our bodies. Unfortunately, physicians are now treating patients who are suffering side effects from taking herbal remedies along with their prescribed medications. This practice can be very dangerous because of very real, negative interactions between herbs and prescribed drugs. Some can be life threatening.

THREE GRADES OF HERBS

There are three basic types of herbs.

Food-grade herbs

Food-grade herbs are taken on a daily basis to support the body, cleanse the system and promote balance. They have a virtually unlimited margin for error, meaning they can be eaten in almost any amount with no reversal of benefits.

Medicinal-grade herbs

Medicinal herbs are used in time of crisis such as cold, flu or infection. These herbs are used for short periods of time for effectiveness. Otherwise, overuse could cause a reversal of benefits to occur.

Poisonous herbs

Poisonous herbs are helpful to bring very short-term, specific benefits, but have no margin for error. If they are misused at all, they will cause a quick and persistent decline in health—and possibly even death.

HERBAL FRIENDS

Your primary goal in using natural remedies for health is to support your body with system-specific nutrition, which will aid the healing process. The following herbal guide will give you information you need to make educated choices when it comes to nourishing, cleansing and strengthening your body with herbs.

Alfalfa

- Eases inflammation; helpful for arthritis
- Acts as a diuretic
- Healing food for digestive disorders
- Lowers cholesterol

Aloe vera

- External uses:
  Antibacterial properties
  Antifungal properties
  Antiviral properties
  Wound and burn healer

- Internal uses:
  Natural laxative
  Soothes stomach
  Helps skin disorders

Astragalus

- Enhances the immune system
- Lowers blood pressure
- Adrenal gland booster
- Provides energy
- Increases metabolism
- Good for battling colds and flu
- CAUTION: Not to be taken when a fever is present

Bilberry

- Strong antioxidant
- Diuretic/urinary tract antiseptic
- Prevents night blindness and cataracts
- May halt macular degeneration
- Helps inflammation
- Useful for anxiety and stress

Black cohosh
- Relieves menopausal hot flashes
- Relieves menstrual cramps
- Helps circulatory and cardiovascular disorders
- Lowers blood pressure
- Reduces cholesterol
- Useful for nervousness and stress
- CAUTION: Do not use during pregnancy.

Black walnut
- Good for eliminating parasites
- Good for fungal infections
- Good for warts and poison ivy
- Aids digestion

Butcher's broom
- Most effective if taken with vitamin C
- Promotes circulation
- Good for varicose veins
- Useful for Ménière's disease
- Good for vertigo

Cascara sagrada
- Natural laxative
- Colon cleanser
- Aids constipation
- Helps in the expulsion of parasites

Cat's claw (uña de gato)
- Antioxidant
- Anti-inflammatory (arthritis)
- Intestinal cleanser
- Helpful for arthritis
- Helpful for tumors (cancer)
- Good for immune system
- CAUTION: Do not use during pregnancy.

Cayenne (capsicum)
- Catalyst for other herbs
- Useful for arthritis and rheumatism (topically and internally)
- Good for colds, flu, sinus infection and sore throat
- Useful for headache and fever
- Aids organs (kidneys, heart, lungs, pancreas, spleen and stomach)
- Improves digestion
- Increases thermogenesis for weight loss

Chamomile (grandma's favorite)
- Helps stress, anxiety and insomnia
- Good for indigestion
- Useful for colitis and most digestive problems

   ❦   CAUTION: Use for short periods of time only. Do not use if you are allergic to ragweed.

Corn silk

   ❦   Wonderful for bladder and kidney health; a natural diuretic
   ❦   Good for edema
   ❦   Helps PMS and prostate disorders

Cranberry

   ❦   Use only unsweetened concentrate or gel capsules
   ❦   Helps acidify the urine, thereby preventing bacteria from adhering to the bladder
   ❦   Prevents urinary tract infections

Damiana

   ❦   Energy tonic
   ❦   Increases libido
   ❦   Brings oxygen to genital region; is an aphrodisiac
   ❦   CAUTION: Interferes with iron absorption; if anemic, use for short term only

Dandelion

   ❦   Great coffee substitute
   ❦   Cleanses liver; increases production of bile
   ❦   Cleanses blood of uric acid and toxins, thereby preventing abscesses, boils and rheumatism
   ❦   Aids kidney, stomach, spleen and pancreas function

Dong quai (angelica)

   ❦   Useful for hot flashes
   ❦   Helpful for PMS
   ❦   Good for menopause
   ❦   Increases ovarian hormones
   ❦   Good for vaginal dryness

Echinacea (coneflower)

   ❦   Boosts white blood cell production
   ❦   Immune system support
   ❦   Has anti-inflammatory and antiviral properties
   ❦   Good for colds, flu and infection
   ❦   CAUTION: Use at first sign of illness, no more than two weeks at a time. Do not use if you are allergic to sunflowers or related species.

Ephedra

   ❦   Central nervous system stimulant
   ❦   Good for allergies, colds, asthma and respiratory conditions
   ❦   Relieves bronchial spasm
   ❦   Decongestant
   ❦   Mood elevator
   ❦   Decreases appetite

❦ CAUTION: Do not use if you have high blood pressure, panic attacks, glaucoma, heart disease, or are taking medication for depression that is a monoamine inhibitor (MAO). Ephedra is not for long-term use.

Eyebright
❦ Good for itchy, allergy eyes
❦ Eye wash for eye irritation

Fenugreek
❦ Natural bulk laxative
❦ Helps asthma and sinus problems (reduces mucus)
❦ Good for lung disorders

Feverfew
❦ Good for fever and headaches
❦ Good for pain and muscle tension
❦ Useful for menstrual problems
❦ CAUTION: Do not use during pregnancy.

Flax
❦ Useful for colon health
❦ Good for bones, skin, teeth and nails
❦ Good for female disorders

Garlic
❦ Helps fight any infection
❦ Detoxifies the body
❦ Enhances immunity
❦ Lowers blood fats
❦ Assists yeast infections
❦ Helps asthma, cancer, sinusitis, circulatory problems and heart conditions
❦ NOTE: Odorless garlic is available (Kyolic by Wakunaga).

Ginger
❦ Helps nausea, motion sickness and vomiting
❦ Useful for circulatory problems
❦ Good for indigestion
❦ Antioxidant
❦ CAUTION: This is a circulatory stimulant.

Ginkgo biloba
❦ Provides mental energy/stimulant
❦ Improves brain health
❦ Improves circulation and oxygen to the brain
❦ Helps memory loss
❦ Good for tinnitis (ringing in the ears)
❦ Increases circulation to relieve cramping
❦ NOTE: Take for at least fourteen days before expecting results.

Ginseng (American, Siberian, Chinese, Korean)
- Good for adrenal gland health
- Enhances immunity
- Helps stress
- Protects against effects of radiation exposure
- Good for fatigue
- CAUTION: Do not use if you have heart disease, low blood sugar or high blood pressure.

Goldenseal
- Natural antibiotic
- Good for inflammation
- Prevents colds, flu and sore throat from developing
- Useful for colon, respiratory, liver, pancreas, spleen and lymphatic health
- Good for disorders of the prostate, vagina, bladder or stomach (infection)
- NOTE: Alternate with echinacea for the best results.
- CAUTION: During pregnancy use only for short periods of time.

Gota kola
- Energizer/central nervous system stimulant
- Diuretic
- Helps heart and liver functions
- Good for depression, fatigue and sleep disorders

Green tea
- Antibacterial
- Contains antimicrobial polyphenols
- Protects against esophageal and oral cancer
- Lessens risk of colon and pancreatic cancer
- Heart health protection
- Promotes fat burning
- CAUTION: Due to the caffeine contained in green tea, limit your intake to two cups daily if you suffer from anxiety or irregular heartbeat.

Hawthorn
- Restores heart muscle
- Helps lower cholesterol
- Aids circulation
- Good for cardiovascular disease; dilates coronary blood vessels

Hops
- Good for anxiety
- Helps nervousness and insomnia
- Helps pain
- Good for ulcers
- Useful for cardiovascular disorders

Horsetail (bottlebrush, shavegrass)

* Good for healthy skin, bones, hair and nails
* Strengthens heart and lungs

Hyssop

* Regulates blood pressure
* Relieves congestion

Kava

* Induces physical and mental relaxation
* Good for stress-related disorders
* CAUTION: Do not drink alcohol with this herb.
* NOTE: May cause drowsiness. Decrease the dosage if this occurs.

Lavender

* Used in aromatherapy as a stress reliever
* Good for depression
* Aids skin health and beauty

Licorice

* Improves adrenal gland function
* Stimulates production of interferon
* Helps asthma, allergies, chronic fatigue, hypoglycemia, fever and bowel function
* CAUTION: Do not use if you are pregnant, have diabetes, glaucoma, high blood pressure, a history of stroke or heart disease. May cause high blood pressure. Use for one week at a time only.

Lobelia

* Aids in the treatment of asthma, colds and bronchitis
* A relaxant
* CAUTION: Do not use for long periods of time. High doses can lower blood pressure and suppress breathing, which can lead to coma.

Marshmallow

* Aids bladder infections
* Diuretic; helps fluid retention
* Helps kidney problems

Milk thistle

* Potent liver protector and stimulant
* Antioxidant
* Protects adrenal glands and kidneys
* Aids bowel disorders

Mullein

* Laxative
* Good for asthma and bronchitis
* Useful for difficulty breathing
* Helps hay fever

Nettle
- Diuretic
- Reduces mucus in lungs
- Expectorant
- Helps allergic disorders

Papaya
- Aids digestion
- Alleviates heartburn and indigestion

Passionflower
- Sedative
- Helps stress-related disorders
- Helps insomnia

Pau d'arco (taheebo, lapacho)
- Antifungal
- Antibacterial
- Antiviral
- Cleanses the blood
- NOTE: Available as a tea. Begin with only one cup daily.

Red clover
- Blood purifier
- Natural antibiotic
- Aids kidney, liver and bowel disorders

St. John's wort
- Aids and relieves depression
- Inhibits viral infections
- CAUTION: Can cause photosensitivity; limit sun exposure.

Saw palmetto
- Good for prostate health
- Inhibits production of DHT to prevent prostate enlargement
- Diuretic and urinary antiseptic

Suma (Brazilian ginseng)
- Immune system booster
- Fights stress and fatigue
- Inhibits certain types of cancer

Tea tree
- Disinfectant
- Antifungal
- Good for vaginitis
- Good for all skin conditions (including acne, insect bites and athlete's foot)
- CAUTION: May irritate skin in sensitive individuals; discontinue use if this occurs.

Turmeric
- Antibiotic, anticancer and anti-inflammatory
- Lowers cholesterol
- Antioxidant

Uva ursi (bearberry)
- Diuretic
- Useful for bladder and kidney infections
- Strengthens heart muscle

Valerian (nature's Valium)
- Aids anxiety, insomnia, fatigue and irritable bowel syndrome
- Good for nervousness and spasms
- Lowers blood pressure
- Sedative

Wild yam
- Aids premenopausal/menopause symptoms (has progesterone-like compounds)
- Relaxes muscles and reduces inflammation
- Aids female disorders: PMS, cramps, etc.

Willow bark (nature's aspirin)
- Helps headache
- Helps backache
- Helps toothache
- Good for sports injuries
- CAUTION: Long-term use may interfere with mineral absorption.

Wormwood
- Useful for vascular disorders
- Expels worms and parasites when combined with black walnut
- Sedative
- CAUTION: Do not use during pregnancy; can cause spontaneous abortion.

Yohimbe
- Aphrodisiac
- Increases libido
- Enhances circulation to the genital region
- Primarily for use by men
- CAUTION: May cause dizziness, high blood pressure, panic attacks and anxiety. Do not use if you have kidney disease.

Yucca
- Aids arthritis
- Purifies the blood
- Helps osteoporosis, osteoarthritis and inflammation

TRY THESE NATURAL REMEDIES INSTEAD OF MEDICATIONS		
CONDITION	MEDICATION	NATURAL REMEDY
Headache	Aspirin, Acetaminophen, Ibupropfen	Feverfew: Take 80 mg Magnesium: Take 400-800 mg daily
Acid stomach	Zantac, Tagamet, Axid, Tums, Maalox	Deglycyrrhizinated Licorice (DGL): Take two 380-mg tablets 20 minutes before meals
Insomnia	Sleeping Pills	Valerian root: Take 150 mg 45 minutes before bedtime
Nasal congestion	Claritin	Quercetin: Take 200 mg 5 minutes before meals
Benign prostatic hyperplasia (BPH)	Proscar	Saw Palmetto: Take 160 mg twice daily

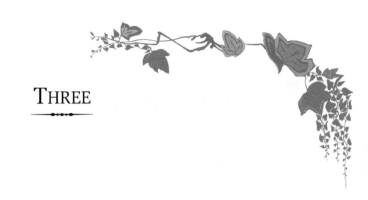

THREE

YOUR TOOLBOX FOR BUILDING HEALTH

C hances are, if you have a handy toolbox at home, you don't use all the tools every day for tasks you need to do. But when the need arises, you automatically go to your toolbox to grab just the right tool you need to finish your task. In the daily task of building and maintaining health, there are many natural tools that you can grab for the help you need. The following recommendations are effective tools you can use to build a solid foundation for a healthy new you.

DETOXIFICATION

"A body with a healthy immune system, efficient organs of elimination and detoxification, and a sound circulatory and nervous system can handle a great deal of toxicity," according to Leon Chaitow, N.D., D.O., of London, England. "But if they have been damaged from chronic exposure to environmental pollutants, restoring these functions, organs, and systems can be accomplished only through detoxification therapies, including fasting, chelation, and nutritional, herbal and homeopathic methods, which accelerate the body's own natural cleansing processes. These therapies will dominate medical thinking in the years ahead."[1]

In my journey toward wellness, detoxification played a large part in my recovery. Detoxification is a way to cleanse our bodies and rid them of toxins and debris that we have accumulated over the years. This gives us a clean foundation upon which we can build. Just like caring for our car engine, filters, hoses and so forth, our bodies need maintenance to promote health. I find it frustrating that people take better care of their cars than they do their physical bodies. Our body's filter—the liver—needs periodic cleansing. We must create a good foundation on which to build our "new," stronger body by doing some internal "house cleaning." This will include what I refer to as changing your filters, cleaning out your cobwebs and tuning up your engine.

Do I need to detoxify?

How do you know if you need to detoxify? There are several indicators. The following symptoms and lifestyles are common in people who are in need of detoxification:

- They suffer from poor elimination.
- They eat a diet of a majority of junk food and sugar.
- They are involved in either overeating, stress eating or late-night eating (or a combination).
- They do not drink sufficient water.
- They suffer from fatigue and stress-related aches, pains and rashes.
- They need antibiotics often.
- Their lifestyle promotes a lack of exercise.
- Other symptoms include insomnia and bad breath.

If you relate to several of these symptoms, detoxification will be a blessing to you and will give you the best start to a stronger immune response. When I began my detoxification process initially, I received a series of six colonic treatments to begin cleansing the colon. I believe these treatments are beneficial but not absolutely essential. If you choose to start your cleansing program in this way, be sure to supplement your intestinal tract with a bowel flora formula such as acidophilus or bifidus. Colonics can strip healthy bowel flora along with the toxins and encrusted matter in the intestines.

If colonic treatments do not appeal to you, try using Nature's Secret Ultimate Cleanse by Lindsey Duncan. (See the product section on page 249.) This formula has been very effective for me, as well as for my family and the hundreds of people with whom I have worked over the past several years. I wish I had access to this product years ago when I struggled with poor bowel function and digestive difficulties. I am delighted with the ease, gentleness and effectiveness of this cleansing product. It involves a two-part program that cleanses all of your channels of elimination, including your liver, kidneys and colon.

If you choose to use Nature's Secret Ultimate Cleanse, it will take about thirty days to consume the two bottles provided in the program. During that time you must drink plenty of nonchlorinated water and eat a diet that is as close to the "garden" as possible—only real food. No preservatives, no refined sugars, cakes, pies, cookies, candy, caffeine, colas, dairy, alcohol or wheat. This cleansing product offers immediate results by gently supporting the body's natural eliminative processes of two to three bowel movements per day. I recommend that you detoxify two times a year—in the spring and fall.

Symptoms to expect when detoxifying

If you have never implemented a detoxification program before, you must know that as your body begins to "clean house" you could develop unpleasant symptoms of headaches, flu, aches and pains, nausea and skin eruptions. These are all positive signs that the cleansing process is working. I always say, "Better out than in," when it comes to toxins! After a few days or weeks on a detoxifying program, your mind will be clear, your energy will soar, you will have better digestion, your skin will glow, and you will sleep better. In essence, you will feel like a new person. After a good detoxification program, you really are a new person!

During this initial phase of detoxification, the energy in the periphery or external parts of your body, such as the muscles and skin, begins to move to the vital internal organs and starts the regeneration and reconstruction process. This shunting of much of the power to the internal region produces a feeling of less energy in the muscles, which the mind interprets as weakness. In actuality, the body's energy is increased, but most of it is being used for rebuilding the important internal organs, which leaves less energy for the muscles.

Be assured that what you are feeling is not true weakness, but a refocusing of energy to the more important internal parts. During this phase it is crucial to not waste energy and to rest and sleep more. This way even more energy can be used for internal regeneration during this crucial phase of detoxification. Do not give in to the temptation to increase your feeling of energy by taking a stimulant of any kind. This will defeat the regeneration process. At first, as you omit toxic substances such as coffee, tea, chocolate, tobacco, excess salt and alcohol, a headache of letdown often occurs. This letdown usually lasts about forty-eight hours and is happily followed by a feeling of well-being and strength.

It is important to be patient with your body and rest in faith that it will accomplish the important task at hand, the cleansing you so desperately need. After a while, you will gain increasing strength, which will far exceed what you felt before you began this makeover program. Your degree of improvement hinges upon your understanding the process at this point. During this deep-cleansing phase determine to rest and relax, limit social obligations and take it easy at work until this "weakness" phase passes.

Renewed energies

As you continue your cleansing process, introducing foods of higher quality while eliminating lower quality foods, remarkable things begin to happen to the body as well as the mind. Did you know that as long as the quality of the food coming into the body is of higher quality than what you used to consume, your body begins to discard the lower grade materials to make room for the new superior materials that are now being consumed? The body will always choose the best materials you give it to make new and healthier tissue. In making our bodies, God designed them to be very selective. The body always tries to produce health and always succeeds unless our interference overwhelms it.

This self-curing nature of the body is evident in many conditions such as the common cold, fevers, cuts, swellings and bruises. These are examples of how the body always strives for health and healing unless we do something to hinder the process.

As you continue, your body will gain more and more energy due to the wonderful live foods that you are consuming in addition to the immune-boosting supplements you have selected. As your body builds up energy, you may experience more unpleasant symptoms. This newly found energy is being used to discard toxic wastes, cellular debris and poisons that cause negative symptoms for a while. It will help to understand that your body is becoming younger and healthier every day because you are throwing off more and more wastes that eventually would have brought pain, disease and much suffering.

I believe that people who have the most bothersome symptoms during their detoxification process, yet continue to follow through to their successful termination, are avoiding some of the worst diseases, which would certainly have developed if they had continued their same unhealthy lifestyle.

Because your body is cyclical in nature, your health will be rebuilt in a series of gradual cycles. You will have good days and not so good days as you journey toward optimal immunity. You will feel better for a few days, and then a set of symptoms will make you feel ill for a couple of days. As you recover, you will feel even better than before. And so goes the process, each set of symptoms gradually becoming milder than the set before them because your body is becoming purer and less toxic each day you commit to the cleansing process.

Your periods of feeling very well become longer and longer and your "symptomatic days" are less and less until you become relatively disease free because your body will be clean and your diet optimal. You will be taking proper supplements for strong immunity and continue to focus on God as your source for healing.

Let faith rise in your heart and become an observer of this healing process. Before your very eyes you will see and feel signs that will cause you to be in awe of God's intelligence at work in your body, mind and spirit.

TIPS FOR DETOXIFICATION

- ❦ Take an acidophilus supplement daily. (I recommend Kyo-Dophilus by Wakunaga.)

- ❦ Buy a loofah, a natural bristle skin brush, and brush your skin (always moving away from the heart) before showering each day This will assist the elimination process for toxins being released through the skin.

- ❦ Drink plenty of pure water, at least six to eight glasses daily.

❧ Include mild exercise such as walking, stretching or bike riding.

❧ Enjoy a salt and soda bath. (See below for instruction on therapeutic baths.)

BATHS FOR PURIFICATION

As I have mentioned, you may experience flu-like symptoms during detoxification because your body is ridding itself of poisons. Relax and soak for a few minutes in one of the therapeutic bath solutions below, and you will feel welcome relief from the unpleasant symptoms you are experiencing.

Before your bath

Skin brushing can be very beneficial because the skin is a primary avenue for detoxification along with the lungs, kidneys, liver and colon. Use a loofah or vegetable brush. You can purchase this at a health food store. You need to brush all parts of the body away from the heart. Then follow this brushing with a sesame oil massage, which will bring a wonderful sense of relief. Massage the whole body for five minutes before bathing or showering.

A Clorox bath

This therapeutic bath will help remove heavy metals from the body and add vital oxygen. Add one-half cup of Clorox brand bleach (use ONLY this brand) to a tub of warm water. Soak for twenty-five minutes. You can shower off with soap and fresh water afterwards if you like, but it is not necessary. If your skin feels a bit itchy, the shower will relieve it.

Epsom salts and ginger

You will open pores and eliminate toxins while also helping to eliminate pain with this bath. Add one cup of Epsom salts and two tablespoons of ginger that has been stirred in a cup of water first to your warm bath. Relax and soak. Do not remain in the tub for more than thirty minutes.

Salt and soda

This bath counteracts the effects of radiation, whether from x-rays, cancer treatment radiation, fallout from the atmosphere or television radiation. Add one cup of baking soda and one to two cups of ordinary coarse salt, Epsom salts or sea salt to a tub of warm water. You can relax and soak for twenty minutes. (More than twenty minutes may exhaust you.)

Epsom-sea-oil

Dry skin and stress can be relieved with this bath. Add one cup of Epsom salts, one cup of sea salt (from health food store) and one cup of sesame oil to a warm to hot tub of water and soak for twenty minutes. Pat yourself dry.

Vinegar bath

This bath is used when the body is too acidic; it is a quick way of restoring the acid-alkaline balance. Add one cup to two quarts of 100 percent apple cider vinegar to a bathtub of warm water. Soak for forty to forty-five minutes. This bath gives excellent relief for joint pain, arthritis, bursitis, tendonitis and gout and is excellent for ridding the body of excess uric acid.

Bentonite bath

Take this bath if you are looking for a fast detoxification method. Soak two to four pounds of bentonite clay in a flat container overnight to dissolve it. Then add the clay to your warm tub of water. If you use two pounds of bentonite, you may soak one hour; with four pounds, you would soak only about thirty minutes. The more bentonite used the faster the detoxification process.

SUGAR SABOTAGE

In times of stress, depression and anxiety, people often reach for their favorite comfort food, which is usually filled with sugar. The long-term consequences of this response are very detrimental to our health, especially to our brain and body functions. In addition, rather than quiet our anxious feelings, excessive sugar consumption will actually increase them.

Results of excessive sugar consumption

Excessive sugar consumption has been shown to suppress our body's immune response, which can lead to disease. For example, if you are consuming too much sugar on a daily basis, you may be setting yourself up for low blood sugar (hypoglycemia). Even small blood sugar fluctuations disturb a person's sense of well-being. Larger fluctuations caused by consuming too much sugar cause feelings of depression, anxiety, mood swings, fatigue and even aggressive behavior.

A study at the University of Alabama showed that people suffering from depression had fewer symptoms when sugar was removed from their diets. Symptoms of anxiety and depression closely parallel many of the symptoms of hypoglycemia: rapid pulse, crying spells, heart palpitations, weakness, cold sweats, irritability, fatigue, nightmares, twitching and poor concentration. If these symptoms are familiar to you, it is possible you are suffering from low blood sugar.

To help restore normal blood sugar levels, you need to focus on eating more fiber and protein foods at each meal and on cutting back on simple sugars. It is very important that you have a protein snack between meals to help keep your blood sugar levels stable all day long.

PERILS OF TOO MUCH SUGAR

MENTAL AND EMOTIONAL SIGNS[2]

  ❧ Chronic or frequent bouts of depression with manic depressive tendencies

  ❧ Difficulty concentrating, forgetfulness or absentmindedness

  ❧ Lack of motivation; loss of enthusiasm for plans and projects

  ❧ Increasing instability, reflected in inconsistent thoughts and actions

  ❧ Moody personality changes with emotional outbursts

  ❧ Irritability, mood swings

BRAIN AND BODY SYMPTOMS

  ❧ Anxiety and panic attacks

  ❧ Bulimia

  ❧ Candidiasis, chronic fatigue syndrome

  ❧ Diabetes or hypoglycemia

  ❧ Food addiction due to stress; B vitamins and minerals are lost as a result of experiencing stress

  ❧ Obesity

  ❧ Menopausal mood swings and unusual low energy

  ❧ High cholesterol and triglycerides, leading to risk of atherosclerosis

  ❧ Excessive food cravings, especially before menstruation

  ❧ Tooth decay and gum loss

Toughing it out!

It is true that eliminating or even limiting sugar will not be easy. But in order to rebuild the health of your brain and body, sugar consumption must be curtailed. By combining low-glycemic foods (like fiber foods) and adding amino acid supplementation and nutritional supplements to help balance your blood sugar, you will optimize your brain biochemistry. The following dietary supplements will be particularly helpful as you make the necessary adjustment of less sugar consumption:

  ❧ Chromium picolinate
  ❧ B-complex

- ❦ Vitamin C
- ❦ Pantothenic acid
- ❦ Adrenal gland supplement
- ❦ Amino acid supplement
- ❦ Calcium and magnesium
- ❦ A protein shake each morning
- ❦ Stevia extract as a sugar-balancing herbal sweetener
- ❦ Increased fiber in your diet (brown rice, for example)

Wisdom for your future

It is wise to make the effort to balance your blood sugar because low blood sugar can predispose you to developing diabetes later in life. Diabetes occurs when the body does not properly utilize the sugar and carbohydrates that a person consumes. Because of years of abuse, the pancreas is no longer able to produce adequate insulin, which creates the condition of high blood sugar. This can be very dangerous. According to the National Institute of Diabetes and Digestive and Kidney Diseases, more than seventeen million people suffer from diabetes in this country.[3] Diabetes can lead to heart and kidney disease, stroke, blindness, hypertension and even death.

Take the short quiz in the chart below to see if your sugar consumption may be affecting your level of health now and if it could lead to serious illness later in life as well. If you answer *yes* to several of these questions, you may need to reconsider your consumption of sugar.

SUGAR CONSUMPTION AND YOUR HEALTH

Yes	No	
❑	❑	Do you have a family history of diabetes?
❑	❑	Do you crave sweets at certain times of the day?
❑	❑	When under stress, do you crave sweets?
❑	❑	Do you consume ice cream, chocolate, pies, cakes and candy more than twice a week?
❑	❑	Do you feel weak and shaky if your meal is delayed?
❑	❑	Do you feel tense, uptight and nervous at certain times during the day?
❑	❑	Do you crave sodas or other sweetened soft drinks?
❑	❑	Do you choose low-fat foods, while ignoring the higher sugar content typically found in them?

No sugar? You've got to be kidding!

If you feel you are addicted to sugar, as many Americans are, you may feel helpless to change your lifestyle so drastically as to eliminate sugar. It is not really difficult. Sugar cravings increase because they deplete the body of necessary elements it needs. For example, you'll be interested to know that people who consume too much simple sugar and who are under constant stress are typically low in chromium. Taking a chromium supplement will help you wean yourself off simple sugars that have been robbing you of your health.

I have often witnessed that my clients experience a heightened sense of well-being after beginning to follow a healthy eating plan and taking chromium picolinate. I have also found that adding chromium to the diet seems to increase energy levels. I believe this is because of the blood sugar balancing effect it exerts on the body. The energy peaks and valleys disappear and are replaced with an evenly sustained energy.

In addition to a chromium supplement, I recommend pantothenic acid, which is a B vitamin that helps the body handle stress. This vitamin does wonders for your adrenal glands, which are so often zapped by caffeine, sugar, stress and lack of sleep. Pantothenic acid and chromium picolinate will help you make the lifestyle changes you need to experience a balanced mind and body.

Instead of sugar, you can learn to use natural whole-food sweeteners discussed on page 30, which will be a wonderful blessing. They are noncaloric and safe for diabetics and hypoglycemics. I urge you to avoid artificial sweeteners, which are as great a risk to your health as too much sugar can be.

Why eliminate artificial sweeteners?

America has jumped on the artificial sweetener bandwagon. This is because of our obsession and preoccupation with our overweight condition. It seems like a simple answer for those trying to watch their sugar calories. However, there are toxic and harmful ingredients in these artificial sweeteners that can damage our health.

Did you know that one of the components of aspartame is methanol? Methanol is considered toxic even in small amounts. In addition, toxic levels of methanol have been associated with brain swelling, inflammation of the heart muscle and the pancreas and even blindness! To help you make your decision regarding aspartame, I recommend that you read *Aspartame (NutraSweet): Is It Safe?* by H. J. Roberts, M.D. (The Charles Press, 1990). This informative book contains reports of convulsions, memory loss, mood swings, headaches, nausea and more that are linked to the consumption of aspartame.

I always tell my clients to eat a diet of foods as close to the original garden as possible. This means eating natural foods that are close to their original form. Aspartame is not natural; it is a synthetic chemical that can harm the body. It is even implicated in fetal brain damage. I encourage pregnant and lactating women, as well as very young or allergy-prone children, to avoid aspartame. There are natural whole-food sweeteners that can satisfy your occasional sweet tooth without risk to your health.

HEALTHFUL SWEETENERS

- **Honey** is a whole food that is twice as sweet as sugar. It also contains vitamins and enzymes. However, you should avoid using honey if you are diabetic or have candida or low blood sugar.

- **Rice syrup,** made from rice and sugar, is 40 percent as sweet as sugar.

- **Sucarat** is a natural sweetener made from sugar cane juice. It is also a concentrated sweetener, like honey, that should be used with caution if you have blood sugar imbalance.

- **Stevia** is a natural sweetener that comes from South America and can be used in beverages, baking and cooking. It is safe for persons with blood sugar imbalances and/or candida and diabetes. Stevia comes in two forms, a liquid extract and a white powered extract.

- **Fructose** is a natural sweetener derived from fruit. It is twice as sweet as sugar and not allowed if you have candida.

A sweet secret

Of the above sweeteners, Stevia is my personal favorite. Stevia is a wonderful tool in weight loss and weight management because it contains no calories, and research indicates it significantly increases glucose tolerance and inhibits glucose absorption. People who ingest Stevia daily often report a decrease in their desire for sweets and fatty foods.

Not only does Stevia add the desired sweetness, but research has also revealed that Stevia effectively regulates blood sugar. This is of vital importance for people who have either high or low blood sugar. In some South American countries Stevia is sold as a helpful aid to people with diabetes and hypoglycemia.

Other studies have demonstrated that Stevia lowers elevated blood pressure but does not seem to affect normal blood pressure adversely. Stevia inhibits the growth and reproduction of some bacteria and other infectious organisms, including the bacteria that cause tooth decay and gum disease. This may help explain why users of Stevia-enhanced products report a lower incidence of colds and flu and why it has such exceptional qualities when used as a mouthwash and toothpaste. Many persons report significant improvement in gum disease following a regular practice of using Stevia.[4]

Other benefits of adding whole-leaf Stevia to the daily diet is that it improves digestion and gastrointestinal function, soothes upset stomachs and helps speed recovery from minor illnesses. An interesting anecdotal claim made by many users is that drinking Stevia tea or Stevia-enhanced teas or placing Stevia leaves in the mouth reduces their desire for tobacco and alcoholic beverages.

Stevia is currently in use as a healthful, no-calorie sweetener in South America, China, Taiwan, Thailand, Korea, Malaysia, Indonesia and Japan. As a sweetener, Stevia in these countries enjoys a 41 percent share of the commercial sugar-substitute market.[5]

GREEN SUPERFOODS

One of the most effective tools for building health is found in the class of foods called green superfoods because they are supercharged with nutrition. It has been said that eating any of these green superfoods is like receiving a little transfusion to enhance immunity and promote energy and well-being. They are one of the richest sources of many essential nutrients. They are nutritionally more concentrated and potent than regular greens like salads and green vegetables. In addition, green superfoods are purposely grown and harvested to maximize and insure high vitamin, mineral and amino acid concentrations. The following list includes green superfoods that are available in most health food stores across the country.

    ❧   **Blue and blue-green algae** are the most potent source of beta carotene available in the world. They are called the perfect superfoods because they are brimming with superior quality proteins, fiber, vitamins, minerals and enzymes.

    ❧   **Spirulina** is extremely high in protein and rich in B vitamins, amino acids, beta carotene and essential fatty acids. It is easy to digest, so it boosts energy quickly and sustains it for long periods of time.

    ❧   **Barley grass** contains vitamins, minerals, proteins, enzymes and chlorophyll. It contains more calcium than cow's milk, vitamin C and B_{12}. It also helps inflammatory conditions of the stomach and digestive system.

    ❧   **Wheatgrass** has been used around the world for many serious diseases to rebuild, cleanse and strengthen the body because of its incredible nutritional value. Fifteen pounds of wheatgrass is equivalent to almost four hundred pounds of the most perfectly grown vegetables.

    ❧   **Kyo-Green** by Wakunaga of America contains barley, wheatgrass, chlorella and kelp. This is a potent formula that helps cleanse the bloodstream, detoxify the system and supply the body with minerals, enzymes and many important nutrients, providing energy for enhanced daily performance.

Kyo-Green is my all time favorite green superfood because of the synergism of the combination of ingredients. I personally use Kyo-Green powder every day. This is what I recommend that you use because of the wonderful formulation of ingredients it provides. Together, the synergism of these ingredients do so much more for your body than any of the green superfoods alone. Try it and feel the difference.

Power Mushrooms

In my quest for wellness years ago, I consumed what I call "power mushrooms." Currently, the interest in these same mushrooms has literally—*mushroomed.* Researchers have found that certain types of mushrooms are filled with a grocery list of substances that may help in fighting disease. The most exciting report is that they boost immunity and that some may be effective against cancer and heart disease. Researchers have discovered that mushrooms produce many beneficial compounds that help their survival against other fungi and microbes.[6]

The same substances that mushrooms use for defense can help humans as well. Mushrooms contain compounds known as polysaccharides. Polysaccharides spark the immune system by helping the body to create T-cells, which are immune system warriors in our bodies that destroy invaders and may halt tumor growth.

It is thought that incorporating any of the power mushrooms into your diet will result in dramatic recoveries because of the synergism they create with your own immune system. According to author Christopher Hobbs in his book *Medicinal Mushrooms,* the chemical steroids and terpenes that mushrooms also contain are thought to help fight the formation of cancerous tumors.[7] By adding one of these power mushrooms to your eating plan, you will be adding one more powerful tool to help build your health. Here are three of the main power mushrooms from God's bounty:

- **Reishi** stimulates immunity, has antitumor properties, is anti-inflammatory and helps to alleviate arthritis.

- **Shiitake** has possible antiviral, anticancer properties and is an energizer. It is also delicious when used in cooking.

- **Maitake** has antitumor properties. It may also protect the liver and lower blood pressure. It contains beta glucans, which are chemicals that boost immunity.[8]

Water Wisdom

Many people in this country suffer from aches and pains, constipation, skin eruptions and fatigue. You may find it hard to believe that a simple lack of water is often behind these common health complaints. Our society consumes coffee by the gallon and soft drinks and iced tea by the liter. Plain old water for some people is just plain boring or worse, distasteful.

Many clients inform me on their first visit that they don't drink water. They assure me that they make sure they drink enough liquids each day. I ask them to tell me what liquids they drink. You guessed it. Iced tea, coffee, concentrated juices and soft drinks! I often see clients who ingest large quantities of vitamin supplements every day with a glass of iced tea or soda! No wonder these people are having problems! Our bodies simply cannot function properly without pure water.

Water makes up 65 to 75 percent of our body. It is second only to oxygen as an essential need for our survival. Water helps to flush wastes and toxins, regulates body temperature and acts as a shock absorber for joints, bones and muscles. It cleanses the body inside and out. It transports nutrients, proteins, vitamins, minerals and sugars for assimilation. When you drink enough water your body works at peak performance. Many of my clients that have a problem with water retention, edema and bloating are simply not drinking enough water. Once they begin to drink adequate water, these symptoms improve. If you are trying to lose weight, you should know that when you drink enough water, your hunger will be curtailed. To maintain the proper function of all of your body's complex systems, you must start drinking good, clean water every day.

The recommended amount of water you need is six to eight glasses per day. If you have not been drinking water and this seems like a lot to you, just start slowly and increase your intake gradually. Add a slice of fresh lemon, and you will get even more of a cleansing benefit. In addition, water is easier to drink with a hint of flavor from a lemon. This works well for my clients who used to believe that they could never increase their water intake. Before long, I see these people out and about with a bottle of water in their hand. It also proves they realize how much better they feel just by drinking enough water; they are so convinced that they carry it with them.

Once people catch the importance of the water idea, the next concern becomes what kind of water you should be drinking. This is a valid concern since most of our tap water is chlorinated, fluoridated or otherwise chemically treated to the point of being an irritant to the system instead of a blessing. Also, many toxic chemicals have found their way into the ground water, adding more pollutants to our water supply.

This growing concern about water purity has led to the huge bottled water industry. Many stores today have whole aisles dedicated to different kinds of bottled water, which can create confusion for the consumer. It may help to clarify the main types of water that are offered. First, there is mineral water, which most often comes from a natural spring with naturally occurring minerals. It has a taste that varies from one spring to the next. Naturally occurring minerals found in mineral water help to aid digestion and bowel function. Europeans have long known the benefits of bottled mineral water. California and Florida regulate the purity of mineral water produced in their states.

Second, there is distilled water. You may have known someone who believes that drinking distilled water is the only way to go. I disagree. While it is true that distilled water is probably the purest water available, it is also de-mineralized. I believe that drinking de-mineralized water on a long-term basis is not ideal. Our bodies need the minerals that naturally occur in water. While distilled water is a good cleanser and detoxifier, I don't believe that it is a good builder because it is devoid of minerals. If you are on a detoxifying program or on chemotherapy, distilled water is excellent to remove debris and toxins. After you are finished with those programs, I advise you to return to drinking a good mineral or spring water to insure proper mineral activity.

Sparkling water is another choice that comes from natural carbonation in underground springs. Most of them are artificially boosted in carbonation by CO_2 to maintain a longer fizz. Many people enjoy sparkling water after dinner as an aid to digestion.

If you choose not to purchase bottled water, you can purify your water by using a water filter in your home. You can purchase water filters that attach to your kitchen sink faucet to remove impurities as water flows out of the tap. You may also have noticed some water pitchers contain filters that purify the water as you fill the pitcher. I feel that these two inventions are quite necessary to help improve the quality of the water we consume. Both options, I feel, are acceptable for health building.

Whatever type of water you choose, the most important thing to remember is that you must pay conscious attention to getting your quota of water every day. Thirst is not a reliable signal that your body needs water. You can easily lose a quart or more of water during activity before you even feel thirsty. Also remember that caffeine and alcohol are diuretics. They increase your body's need for water. If you consume caffeine or alcohol, please make sure you drink enough water to compensate. Ideally, caffeine and alcohol do not belong in a health-building program.

In addition to making sure that your water intake is optimal, it will be helpful to consider your need to take the time to quench your spiritual thirst. Jesus referred to this need when He declared:

> Whosoever drinketh of the water that I shall give him shall never thirst; but the water that I shall give him shall be in him a well of water springing up into everlasting life.
>
> —JOHN 4:14, KJV

WATER FILTERS			
FILTER TYPE	COST	HOW IT WORKS	HARMFUL ELEMENTS REDUCED
Distillation	$800–4,500 whole house system $100–1,000 countertop model $600–1,100 free-standing unit	Boils water, creating a water vapor that leaves contaminants behind. This purified water vapor is then condensed to a liquid.	chromium, lead, nitrates, sulfate, giardia, arsenic, cadmium

| | WATER FILTERS | | |
FILTER TYPE	COST	HOW IT WORKS	HARMFUL ELEMENTS REDUCED
Reverse osmosis (known as "RO" Water)	$600–1500 under-the-counter model $150–200 countertop model	Forces pressurized water through a purifying membrane that eliminates contaminants; purified water then goes to a holding tank.	radium, chromium, iron, cadmium, color, chlorine, lead, radium, giardia, sulfate
Carbon Filtration	$350-up under-the-counter model $25–$30 faucet model	Water passed through a carbon or charcoal block, which traps contaminants; filters must be replaced periodically	chlorine, odors, chemicals, pesticides, bad taste
Water Softener	$1000-3,500	Uses sodium (rock salt) to "soften" the water	Calcium, radium, iron

ANTIOXIDANTS

Essential tools for building a healthy body are antioxidants, which are powerful immune boosters. Our body's immune system protection consists of macrophages, white blood cells, antibodies, lymphatic tissue and the thymus gland. In recent years, science has uncovered health-destroying substances called free radicals that attack our body's defenses, weakening them so that they cannot properly protect us.

Free radicals damage healthy cells. The good news is that they can be subdued by antioxidants that neutralize the harmful free radicals, thereby preventing the weakening and damaging of our cells. There are three basic sources of free-radical activity. First, free radicals are formed as by-products during exercise, illness and by taking certain medications. Second, they are caused by air pollution, smoke, radiation and pesticides. Third, free radicals form other free radicals.

Antioxidants come to the rescue. Their job is to travel the bloodstream and localize in our cells and organs, locating and neutralizing free radicals. After they neutralize or quench these free radicals, the antioxidants become inactive and are eliminated from the body. This means we must continually supply our bodies with needed antioxidants, either through the foods we eat, by taking supplements or both.

The four major antioxidants are pro-vitamin A (or beta carotene), vitamin C, vitamin E and selenium. These antioxidant nutrients provide a four-point attack. Pro-vitamin A, or beta carotene, quenches singlet oxygen molecules, vitamin C protects tissues and blood components, vitamin E protects cell membranes, and selenium is a vital part of antioxidant enzymes. All together, these powerful four "mop up" free radicals as they form and before they do their damage to our system.

I personally use and recommend Carlson ACES as my formula of choice for antioxidant protection. Their formula contains pro-vitamin A, or beta carotene (10,000 IU), vitamin C in a nonacidic calcium ascorbate form (1,000 mg), vitamin E in the form of natural d-alpha tocopherol (400 IU) and selenium (100 mcg). The dose is two soft gel capsules daily. (See product information at the end of the book.)

To recap, it is important that we understand that free radicals can destroy our health by damaging healthy cells. Antioxidants defend us against free-radical activity.

JUICING

By now, many of you may have heard about juicing and how beneficial it is for your body. Thanks to the popular JuiceMan juicer, millions of Americans have heard about juicing and the incredible amount of nourishment it gives to our body.

Why is reducing fresh fruits and raw vegetables to juice in special combinations so health promoting? Because drinking these fresh juices extracted from raw fruits and vegetables furnishes all the cells in the body with the elements they need in a manner in which they can be easily and quickly assimilated.

Fruit juices are the cleansers of our bodies, and vegetable juices are the builders and regenerators of our systems. Vegetable juices contain all the minerals, salts, amino acids, enzymes and vitamins that the human body requires. This is why both fruit and vegetable juices are so important.

Another benefit of adding juices to your diet is that juices are digested and assimilated within ten to fifteen minutes after consumption. They are then utilized almost completely by the body to nourish and regenerate the cells, tissues, glands and organs. The end result is very positive because of the minimal effort needed by the digestive system to assimilate them.

One of the most important things to remember about juicing is to drink your juices fresh daily. That is when they are at their peak as far as nutritional value. Also, fresh juices spoil quickly, so it is better to make fresh juice daily. In addition, if you are ill or have a history of digestive difficulty, be sure to dilute your juice with water in a fifty-fifty mix. This way you will prevent any bloating, gas or other discomfort you could experience from ingesting this powerful liquid nutrition into your body. Another important consideration is to drink fruit juices at different times of the day than vegetable juices in order to prevent stomach upset.

As a general rule of thumb, one pint daily is the least amount needed to experience positive results. When I was eating therapeutically to regain my health, I drank two or three pints of fresh fruit and vegetable juices daily.

I have included some of the same juice combinations that I have personally used and ones that I have recommended to my clients for various sub-health conditions. I recommend that you wash the fruits and vegetables in ten drops of grapefruit seed extract in a basin of water. This washing will kill yeast, mold and fungi. In addition, grapefruit seed extract is a disinfectant. Be sure to scrub the fruits and vegetables with a brush to help remove any pesticide residue.

FRESH JUICE FORMULAS

CONDITION	JUICES
Arthritis	Grapefruit
	Carrot and spinach
	Celery
	Carrot and celery
Anemia	Carrot, celery, parsley and spinach
	Carrot and spinach
	Carrot, beet and celery
Bladder trouble	Carrot and spinach
	Carrot, beet and cucumber
	Carrot, celery and parsley
Bronchitis	Carrot and spinach
	Carrot and dandelion
	Carrot, beet and cucumber
Colds	Carrot, beet and cucumber
	Carrot, celery and radish
	Carrot and spinach
Constipation	Carrot and spinach
	Spinach
	Carrot
Fatigue	Carrot
	Carrot and spinach
	Carrot, beet and cucumber

Fresh Juice Formulas	
CONDITION	**JUICES**
Fever	Grapefruit Lemon Orange
Gallbladder and gallstones	Carrot, beet and cucumber Carrot and spinach Carrot, celery and parsley
Headaches	Carrot and spinach Carrot, celery, parsley and spinach Carrot, lettuce and spinach
Insomnia	Carrot and spinach Carrot and celery Carrot, beet and cucumber
Liver problems	Carrot, beet and cucumber Carrot and spinach Carrot
Menopausal symptoms	Carrot and spinach Carrot, beet, lettuce and turnip
Nervous tension	Carrot and spinach Carrot and celery Carrot, beet and cucumber
Sciatica	Carrot and spinach Carrot, spinach, turnip and watercress
Sinus trouble	Carrot and spinach Carrot, beet and cucumber Carrot
Ulcers	Carrot and spinach Carrot, beet and cucumber Cabbage

TOP TEN LIFE-ENHANCING SUPPLEMENTS

Another set of tools you will find very effective in building your healthy body include the following ten life-enhancing supplements. Consider the brief description of their function and learn to use them as needed to strengthen your personal health.

Creatine

Creatine provides safe nutritional support for athletes seeking peak performance in short-duration, high-intensity workouts. Creatine supports the body's natural ability to regenerate the primary energy immediately available to working muscle. This supplement has the potential to increase optimal work output in activities such as weight training and running.

Suggested dose: Up to 20 grams daily, mixed with juice or water. After you achieve the desired results, go on the maintenance dose of 5–15 grams daily in divided doses.[10]

Conjugated linoleic acid (CLA)

Usually derived from sunflower oil, CLA has been shown to play an important role in reducing body fat and increasing muscle retention. It was developed and patented by scientists at the University of Wisconsin's Food Research Institute. CLA improves cell metabolism, which helps the body reduce fat levels and increase muscle retention. Because of the way our foods are raised and produced, the amount of CLA we receive in our diet is lowered from previous years. This is one reason that Americans are seeing a substantial increase in body fat levels.

Suggested dose: Two 500-mg capsules before each meal.[11]

Pregnenolone

Pregnenolone, known as the well-being hormone, is a natural precursor to over one hundred fifty steroid hormones. It helps to support the immune system, mood and memory. Studies show that the body makes 60 percent less pregnenolone at age seventy-five than it does at age thirty-five. In the body, supplemental pregnenolone takes one or two metabolic pathways, converting to DHEA and/or progesterone. Pregnenolone has been shown to convert appropriately according to body's needs.

Suggested dose: One 10-mg capsule with a meal daily. *Do not take if you are pregnant or lactating.*[12]

5-HTP

5-hydroxytryptophan (5-HTP) is an intermediate in the natural synthesis of the essential amino acid tryptophan to serotonin. 5-HTP is derived from the *Griffonia Simplicifolia* plant and is an important neurotransmitter involved in the regulation of brain activity responsible for emotion, appetite and wake/sleep/wake cycles. By feeding your brain 5-HTP, your serotonin level rises, which in turn causes emotional well-being, appetite control and better sleep quality.

The signs of serotonin deficiency include depression, anxiety, panic attacks, migraine headaches, PMS, insomnia, obesity, fibromyalgia, alcoholism, OCD (obsessive compulsive disorder), chronic pain, hyperactivity, mood swings and aggressive or violent behavior.

Suggested dose: 50-mg capsule once a day before a meal. *Do not use if you are pregnant or lactating.*[13]

Resveratrol

Resveratrol promotes cardiovascular health by its antioxidant action and its ability to modulate platelet aggregation and arachidonic acid metabolism. Resveratrol is a compound that is often associated with the health benefits of red wine because of its powerful antioxidant and cardio-protective properties. It is derived from *Polygonum cuspidatum,* an herb that has been used for centuries for its nutritional benefits.

Suggested dose: 200-mg capsule daily.[14]

Chitosan

Chitosan provides a natural way to influence fat digestion and to maintain healthy cholesterol levels. Derived from chitin, chitosan dissolves into a gelled form that traps fat in the intestines and helps inhibit its absorption. It appears to decrease the primary enzyme of cholesterol synthesis and has demonstrated the ability to promote higher levels of beneficial HDL cholesterol.

Suggested dose: 250 mg four times daily in divided doses.[15]

Coenzyme Q_{10}

Coenzyme Q_{10} is a necessary component of cellular energy production and respiration. It enhances energy levels in every cell of the body, providing increased energy and exercise tolerance and optimal nutritional support of the cardiovascular system. It is especially supportive of tissues that require a lot of energy such as periodontal tissue, the heart muscle and the cells of the body's defense system.

Suggested dose: Two to four capsules per day in divided doses with meals. Take with vitamin E for enhanced benefit.[16]

Olive leaf extract

Derived from the Mediterranean olive tree, olive leaf extract is popular in herbal and folk remedies and has benefited mankind for over one hundred fifty years. Oleuropein, the active nutrient in olive leaf, is a powerful foe against bacteria, fungi, parasites and yeast. Olive leaf provides natural protection and a healthy environment for cells without suppressing immune system function or harming beneficial microflora.

Suggested dose: One to two capsules of standardized extract (500 mg) in divided doses, between meals.[17]

Melatonin

Produced by the pineal gland, melatonin is a hormone that regulates the body's wake/sleep/wake cycle. The hormone is secreted in a circadian rhythm by enzymes, which are activated by darkness and depressed by light. Nightly melatonin supplementation can boost the performance of immune systems that are compromised by age, drugs or stress during sleep.

Suggested dose: One 3-mg capsule one-half to one hour before bedtime. *Do not take if you are pregnant or lactating.*[18]

Phosphatidylserine

Phosphatidylserine is found in all cells, but it is most heavily concentrated in brain cells. This brain nutrient improves cognitive function, emotional

well-being and behavioral performance by restoring cell membrane composition. Mental acuity is positively affected by supplementation with
phosphatidylserine.

Suggested dose: Three 100-mg capsules daily in divided doses with meals.[19]

PROBIOTICS: GASTROINTESTINAL DEFENDERS

If you are battling any kind of digestive or intestinal problem, probiotics
(good bacteria) are a must for your health-building toolbox. These gastrointestinal defenders are crucial in keeping your immune defense in good
working order. They consist mainly of lactobacillus acidophilus and lactobacillus bifidus. They produce volatile fatty acids, which provide metabolic
energy. In addition, they help you digest food and amino acids, produce certain vitamins and, most importantly, make your lower intestine mildly
acidic, thus inhibiting the growth of bad bacteria such as *E. coli*, which has
caused serious illnesses in recent years.

Probiotic supplementation is absolutely essential in your fight against candida or any fungal infection because of the antifungal properties that these
defenders possess. According to Dr. James F. Balch in his best-selling book
Prescription for Nutritional Healing, the flora in a healthy colon should consist of at least 85 percent lactobacilli and 15 percent coliform bacteria.[20] The
typical colon bacteria count today is the reverse, which has resulted in gas,
bloating, intestinal and systemic toxicity, constipation and malabsorption of
nutrients, making it a perfect environment for the overgrowth of candida. By
adding probiotics, that is, lactobacillus acidophilus and lactobacillus bifidus
supplements, to your system, you will return your intestinal flora to a
healthier balance and eliminate all of the problems of intestinal flora imbalance mentioned.

If you are on antibiotic therapy, it is vitally important that you supplement
your digestive tract with probiotics (good bacteria) because antibiotic use
destroys your healthy bowel flora along with the harmful bacteria. Both lactobacillus acidophilus and lactobacillus bifidus promote proper digestion,
help to normalize bowel function and prevent gas and candida overgrowth.
This in turn keeps immunity high.

Store your probiotic formula in a cool, dry place. Some brands require
refrigeration. I personally prefer and use Kyo-Dophilus from Wakunaga of
America because it is milk free and remains viable and stable even at high
temperatures. It contains 1.5 billion live cells per capsule, is suitable for all
ages and contains lactobacillus acidophilus, B. bifidum and B. longum in a
vegetable starch complex. In addition, it is free of preservatives, sugar,
sodium, yeast, gluten, artificial colors and flavors and, as mentioned, milk.

As a dietary supplement, take one capsule with a meal twice daily. Children
under four should take one-half capsule with a meal twice daily. If the child
cannot swallow the capsule, simply open it and sprinkle it in juice or on food.

Natural Antibiotics

There are many natural substances that are powerful antibiotics.

Biotic silver

Biotic silver (pure silver protein) is a very powerful natural antibiotic and antifungal solution that is so effective that it kills and removes from the body all bacteria, viruses and fungi within a short period of time. According to Gary Carlson, director of the Candida Wellness Center in Provo, Utah, this natural antibiotic is extremely effective and overcomes serious infections. It has been approved by the Food and Drug Administration and is classified as a dietary mineral supplement. There are no side effects recorded in decades of use, and studies at the University of Toronto concluded that no toxicity, even in high dosages, results from using biotic silver.

Having sufficient pure silver protein in the body is like having a superior second immune system. Long ago, when the earth was more fertile and our food supply was purer and more natural, there was more silver in the soil, and it would be absorbed into our food. This silver would prevent infectious disease because no yeast, bacteria or virus can survive in the presence of silver. But today, due to the mining of silver for its monetary value and the inorganic methods of farming, there is little silver left in the soil. In addition, strains of infectious organisms are so much stronger today that larger than normal amounts of silver are necessary to eradicate them.

Research indicates that biotic silver protein has been used successfully in the treatment against more than six hundred fifty diseases. These include allergies, athlete's foot, pneumonia, pleurisy, bladder infections, boils, candida and yeast infections, cold sores, cold, flu, cystitis, dermatitis, fungal infection, indigestion, lupus, lyme disease, malaria, psoriasis, rhinitis, ring worm, sinus infections, staph, tonsillitis, viruses of all forms (including staph and strep), warts and whooping cough. And it helps prevent disease as well.

Biotic silver is the most advanced form of colloidal silver for the therapeutic purpose of fighting infection available today. The superior effect comes from a special scientific process that allows it to reach negative microorganisms quickly and destroy them completely everywhere in the body. Once the pure silver protein has accomplished its goal of eradicating disease, it is removed from the body with no toxic accumulation or side effects.

Silver particle size is important when it comes to a superior silver protein formula. In the case of biotic silver, it is certified to have silver particles down to .001 microns or smaller, which allows the particles to flow freely through even the smallest capillaries of the body and enter and be removed completely from the cells and tissues. It is a product that is well designed and formulated from the finest research and scientific achievements in the fields of parasitology and probiotics.

Biotic silver can even be given to infants and can be used during pregnancy. Because it is a special proprietary formulation, it does no harm to human enzymes, hormones or any part of the body chemistry. Tests in hospitals, universities and research laboratories over decades have proven this beyond a doubt. No one has ever overdosed, and it is not an allopathic poison.

Biotic silver is gold in color, tasteless, odorless and does not upset the stomach. It is nontoxic, nonaddictive, nonaccumulative and completely safe. (For ordering information, see the product section on page 249.)

Olive leaf extract

Olive leaf is a 100 percent natural herbal antibacterial, antiviral and anti-fungal extract taken from specific parts of the olive tree. In addition, it is a nontoxic immune system builder. Olive leaf may also be a potent tool against the common cold and flu. Other benefits that researchers have found is that olive leaf could lower blood sugar, rid people of bladder infections, asthma, swollen glands, scalp and skin conditions, sinus infections and more.

Recently a more concentrated form of olive leaf extract has been developed and is marketed under the name of Defend. Several long-term sufferers of chronic fungal infections have noticed regression or clearing faster when they used Defend than when they used another product. According to Gary Carlson, many individuals with fibromyalgia, Epstein-Barr virus, long-term infections and chronic fatigue syndrome are reporting that they feel much better and have more complete relief when taking Defend.

Goldenseal

Goldenseal acts as an antibiotic and has anti-inflammatory and antibac-terial properties. It is good for any infectious disease. If you use it at the first sign of cold, flu or sore throat, it may stop it from developing at all. If it doesn't stop it completely, it will shorten the duration of the symptoms.

Oil of oregano

Oil of oregano is a very powerful antibacterial agent. Use it very sparingly.

Grapefruit seed extract

Grapefruit seed extract is antifungal, antibacterial and antiviral. It is avail-able in a liquid or capsule form. Nasal sprays are also available.

FOCUS ON FATS

For optimum health, it is important to focus on the right kind of fats. I'm talking about fatty acids that are so necessary for good health that they are called essential fatty acids (EFAs). Essential fatty acids will have a positive effect on many systems of your body. If you are focusing on candida eradica-tion, you should know that essential fatty acids are beneficial in candida removal and system regeneration process.

EFAs help to improve the texture and condition of your skin and hair; they aid in arthritis prevention and treatment; they help to lower cholesterol and triglyceride levels and help lower blood pressure. They also help alleviate psoriasis and eczema and are crucial in nerve impulse transmission in the brain, thereby improving brain function. EFAs are used by our bodies in the production of prostaglandins, which act as regulators and messengers of certain body processes.

How important are EFAs? All living cells need essential fatty acids. There are two main types of EFAs. The first is called omega-3, which can be found in deep-water fish like salmon, mackerel and sardines, as well as in canola oil and, my favorite, flaxseed oil. The second type of EFAs is called omega-6, which can be found in grape seed oil, sesame oil, vegetable oil, soybean oil, seeds, nuts and legumes.

When it comes to supplementation, there are several ways to go. First, you may add any of the abovementioned food sources to your eating plan to insure adequate EFA intake, or you may use the following supplements that I have found to be very good in clinical use.

EFAs Supplements	
Omega-3	Flaxseed oil capsules or liquid can aid arthritis relief and lower cholesterol and triglyceride level.
	Carlson Salmon Oil liquid or capsules are excellent for arthritis.
Combination omega-3 and omega-6	Nature's Secret Ultimate Oil (follow directions on label)
	Wakunaga's Kyolic EPA (follow manufacturer's directions on dosage)

Use only olive oil when you cook. Olive oil reduces the amount of LDL in the bloodstream. It has been said that incorporating olive oil in your diet can lower your LDL levels better than eating a low-fat diet. In order for cholesterol levels to drop, however, you must add fiber in addition to olive oil and your EFA-combination omega-3 and omega-6 formula.

Please note that even though you will find most of your natural oils in dark containers to keep out light, keeping them in the refrigerator and using them up quickly will insure they don't become rancid, because they can go rancid quickly. If you cannot use a bottle of oil up in a month, then purchase a smaller bottle. This is especially true if you choose flaxseed oil. I keep my combination Nature's Secret Ultimate Oil or Kyolic EPA in my refrigerator even though it is not imperative that you do so. When you supplement your system with essential fatty acids or oils, your body truly runs like a "well-oiled" machine.

Enzymes for Improved Immune Function

Enzymes are crucial. This is because they turn the foods that we eat into energy and unlock this energy for use in the body. Our bodies make two basic types of enzymes: digestive and metabolic. Our bodies secrete enzymes to help us break down food into nutrients and wastes. These enzymes include pepsin, lipase, protease, amylase, trypsin and ptyalin. We also receive enzymes from raw foods (juicing promotion) that we eat and also by taking enzyme supplements. The strength of our enzyme activity is important in building a stronger immune system as well as healthier blood.

In our busy lifestyles and hectic schedules, we overcook, microwave and overprocess our foods, killing all or most of the enzymes. While it's true that we occasionally eat raw foods that do contain live enzyme activity, our consumption of cooked "dead enzyme" foods is greater. This leaves our bodies the big job of producing more enzymes to break down these cooked foods. That is, unless we supplement.

I have seen people gain more energy, lose weight, sleep better and feel better in general after simply beginning to supplement their bodies with enzymes. This is because our bodies work more efficiently with proper enzyme activity. No excess energy has to be expended by the body on the process of digestion. It has been said that we are only as healthy as what we assimilate and eliminate. After awhile you will assimilate or digest more effectively with the help of supplemental enzymes, and you will experience better elimination by detoxifying your body.

A variety of supplemental enzymes are available. It is very important that you use an enzyme supplement tailored to your particular situation. Also, you must make sure that the doses are measured in active units, which are the most potent.

In my research, I found that there are four basic types of enzyme deficiencies:

- A lack of protease limits your ability to digest proteins.
- A lack of lipase hampers your ability to digest fats.
- A deficiency of amylase affects your ability to digest carbohydrates.
- A deficiency of any two or more enzymes can lower the quality of your life because of lowered immune response.

Enzymes have far-reaching benefits. They deliver nutrients, carry away toxic wastes, digest food, purify the blood, deliver hormones by feeding and fortifying the endocrine system, balance cholesterol and triglyceride levels, feed the brain and cause no harm to the body.

If we fortify the endocrine system, get the bowels working regularly and digest our food with the help of enzymes (preventing it from turning to fat), we can be truly successful at losing weight and gaining energy. Younger-looking skin is an additional benefit of proper enzyme supplementation. Enzymes can fight the aging process by increasing the blood supply to the skin, delivering life-giving nutrients and then carrying away waste products that can make your skin look old, tired and wrinkled. Because circulation slows down as we age, enzyme supplementation becomes crucial as we grow older.

Now, the question is what type of enzymes do you need to digest food? By enzyme supplementation we want to help the body complete the digestive process without overstressing the body's enzyme-making potential. We will then be in a much more favorable position to fight biological and system malfunctions while boosting our immune system to a higher level.

I have been very pleased with the enzyme formulations I have used from Enzymedica of Punta Gorda, Florida. I have found the following four formulas to be extremely effective personally and in clinical use. The first formula is called *Digest*. This formula speeds digestion of food while reducing the body's need to produce digestive enzymes. Take one capsule with each meal. One capsule is usually sufficient for alleviating poor digestion. If you are in poor health, you may need two to five capsules until your digestion improves. Digest contains high-potency multiple enzymes along with lactobacillus acidophilus to help maintain healthy bowel flora. This formula helps you to digest protein, starch, fat, sugar and fiber.

The second formula is *Purify*. It contains the highest available potency of protease to help digest protein invaders in the blood. This would include parasites, fungal infections, bacteria and viruses, which are covered by a protein film. The enzyme protease breaks down the undigested protein, toxins and debris in the blood, thereby unburdening the immune system so it can concentrate its full action. The recommended dosage is three capsules first thing in the morning and right before bed. This formula is excellent for candida sufferers who traditionally have difficulty with protein digestion and tend to have a toxic load in their bloodstream.

The third formula is *Lypo*. This is an excellent formula that contains the highest available potency of lipase, which digests fats in the blood and digestive tract. This will help to lower cholesterol and triglycerides. It provides additional support for digestion of carbohydrates and dairy products and aids elimination. The recommended dosage is two capsules with each meal. If you are overweight, meaning more than twelve pounds over your ideal weight, the dosage is three capsules with meals. People who are obese are usually low in lipase.

Gastro is the last formula on my list of super enzymes. This formula helps to soothe the gastrointestinal system and alleviate abdominal discomfort. This formula helps to relieve the burning and irritation that some people experience with digestion.

You can see that enzymes can greatly improve your life. According to DicQie Fuller Ph.D., D.Sc., author of *The Healing Power of Enzymes,* it is almost certain that an enzyme depletion exists anytime we suffer from an acute or chronic illness![21] I highly recommend that you add her book to your library if you want to learn more about enzymes. I call enzymes God's sparks of life.

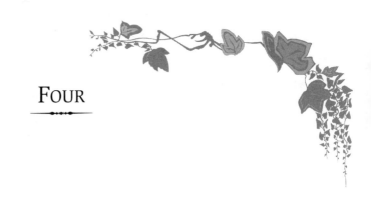

FOUR

NATURAL HEALING PROTOCOLS

The following natural healing protocols enable you to be proactive when it comes to health. Studies have shown that when a person takes an active part in their wellness protocol, healing is swifter, more successful and complete.

TAKING RESPONSIBILITY

Persons who rely solely upon their physician for their wellness are often expecting too much. You have to take at least a measure of responsibility for your own health. These are several of the most widely used natural healing modalities.

Massage

Massage aids in relaxation, gives relief from pain and provides increased range of motion. There is an increasing demand these days for therapeutic massage. It is part of a huge trend toward healthcare with a mind, body and spirit approach. Massage is one modality used to keep the body healthy, promoting relaxation and stress reduction. Massage therapy has become an integral part of healthcare used in the offices of orthopedic doctors, chiropractors and physical therapists. It is well known that stress is one of the primary causes of illness. Massage helps to release both stored physical and emotional tension.

Massage is the systematic and scientific manipulation of the soft tissues of the body. Manipulations fall into four general categories: compressing, vibrating, percussing and gliding.

Massage physiologically relieves pain and metabolically prepares the injured or involved muscles for exercise or movement to their fullest capacity.

In addition, massage can be used to prepare healthy muscles for sports activity or to aid in recovery after a sports activity. For thousands of years massage has been used to relieve pain. It is a useful part of the healing process and is a viable health discipline. Research supports the following:

    ❧   Massage improves blood circulation throughout the body.

    ❧   Deep tissue and lymphatic drainage massage is a wonderful detox-ification therapy, promoting elimination and drainage of mucus and fluid from the lungs.

    ❧   Massage helps relieve headaches.

    ❧   Massage helps to break up adhesions and scar tissue.

    ❧   Massage aids digestive disorders, chronic fatigue, cardiovascular disorders and gynecological problems.

There are five popular types of massage. You may select the method that most suits your physical need.

POPULAR TYPES OF MASSAGE

Swedish massage	Swedish massage involves kneading, friction, tapping and stroking to relax and cleanse the body. It helps muscles, nerves, joints and the endocrine system. It stimulates the body's circulation and will speed healing from injury.
Alexander massage	Alexander massage works to improve posture, expand the chest cavity, improve breathing and body movement.
Feldenkrais	Feldenkrais helps people to change the way they move and change unbalanced muscle patterns through body manipula-tion and exercise.
Rolfing	Rolfing is deep manipulating of connective tissue.
Polarity	Polarity is based on the human body's magnetic field. The magnetic current and movement pattern is accessed to release blocks.

Massage can be used to prevent, treat and heal many conditions. However, massage is not recommended in cases of cancer, high fever, infec-tion, high blood pressure, phlebitis, varicose veins, diabetes, broken bones, cysts or bruises. In addition, use caution with swollen limbs, employing gentle massage only above the swelling.

Hydrotherapy

Hydrotherapy is the practice of using hot or cold water therapeutically to improve many conditions, including stress, arthritis, headaches, menstrual problems, muscle pain, asthma and back pain.

Osteopathy

Osteopathy is similar to chiropractic treatment, focusing on treating mechanical problems of the skeletal system. It is an effective treatment for many conditions, including osteoarthritis, back pain, breathing problems, digestive problems, strain from sports injuries, sciatica and stress.

Reflexology

This technique involves manipulating reflex points on the hands or feet that correspond to different organ systems of the body. It helps to control pain and promote well-being. Reflexology is useful especially in the following conditions: liver problems, kidney disorders, heart disease, digestive complaints, menstrual problems, sinusitis and stress.

Myotherapy

This therapy treats muscles by using manual or electrical stimulation of trigger points in order to relieve pain. It is very effective in treating chronic musculoskeletal pain, sports injuries and TMJ.

Macrobiotic diet

This therapeutic diet involves the use of brown rice and specific vegetables to rebalance the body, to help heal degenerative disease and to promote health. Macrobiotic diet therapy has been used extensively for cancer, arthritis, stress, digestive disorders and depression.

Orthomolecular therapy

This therapy uses vitamins therapeutically. This means larger doses are used to treat specific diseases such as cancer, diabetes, aging, high blood pressure, colds, flu, PMS, menopause and more.

Light therapy

Light therapy is used in the treatment of seasonal affective disorder (SAD), depression and anxiety. It involves the use of sunlight or light boxes to lift mood.

Acupressure

Acupressure involves pressing certain points on the body in order to relieve pain and remove circulatory blockages, thereby reestablishing flow or light force commonly known as *chi* in Chinese medicine. It is very effective for the relief of back pain, muscle pain, head and neck aches and in respiratory problems like asthma. This technique is thousands of years old.

Acupuncture

This technique is similar to acupressure, but uses very fine needles placed strategically along meridians that correspond to different nerves, muscles or organs. It is really quite painless and is remarkable in the fact that it can either stimulate or sedate any area of the body to rebalance the *chi*. Much success has been shown over thousands of years in the treatment of headaches, back pain, liver and kidney problems, smoking, insomnia, allergies, anxiety, depression and much more. Some people go a few times a year for a "tune up" even before they demonstrate symptoms. Again, preventative maintenance is much better than scrambling for a cure.

Colonic therapy

Colonics involve the insertion of a small hose into the rectum, which then sends water throughout the entire length of the colon to gently clean out toxins. Usually done in a series of four to six sessions, colonic therapy has been very successful in the treatment or alleviation of constipation, diverticulitis, candida overgrowth and more.

Chiropractic

Also known as joint manipulation therapy, chiropractic is very effective in treating stress-related pain, muscular pain, injury pain, sciatica and more by adjusting subluxations that occur throughout the entire skeletal system.

Homeopathy: "Like cures like"

Homeopathy is a very gentle two-hundred-year old system of healing that uses extremely diluted medicines or remedies that are designed to activate the body's own healing ability. The remedies are derived from minerals, plants or animals. A homeopathic remedy delivers a tiny amount of a substance that if taken in larger amounts would produce the same symptoms associated with the ailment being treated.

It has been said that a good way to begin a natural healing program is with homeopathic medicine. Once the body's electrical activity is stimulated by the gentle remedy, other natural therapies become even more effective. Homeopathic remedies act as catalysts for the immune system to eradicate the root cause of a particular illness. Studies have shown that homeopathic remedies can reduce the need for antibiotic therapy and other drugs that have risks and side effects. Homeopathic remedies can be used within the following three contexts: prevention of illness, support during illness and recovery or restoration of health.

I have included the ten most popular homeopathic remedies in Appendix A. For more information on homeopathy, contact the National Center for Homeopathy, 801 N. Fairfax, Alexandria, VA 22314.

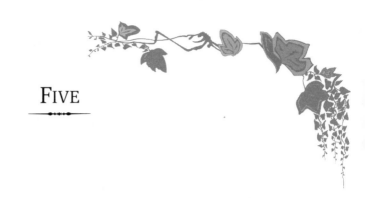

FIVE

NATURE'S NATURAL THERAPIES

I want to introduce you to Bach Flower Essences, a natural method of establishing equilibrium and emotional harmony through the use of wild flowers. When a few drops of specially formulated essences are ingested or rubbed on the skin, they display remarkable healing power.

A MEDICAL PIONEER

Edward Bach, a medical doctor and bacteriologist, gave up his lucrative practice to study the emotional link to ill health in the early 1900s. He believed that if a patient's emotional balance was corrected, the body's natural God-given ability to throw off illness would be strengthened. In the 1930s, Dr. Bach began to search for simpler, more natural medications than the vaccines he had previously formulated. He found his natural medicines in the wild flowers growing around the pastoral cottage he maintained in Oxfordshire, England.

Dr. Bach is recognized as a pioneer in the field of mind-body medicine. He began to recognize that certain types of people (personalities) reacted mentally and emotionally in similar ways to particular diseases. His studies led him to divide people into seven categories and to diagnose them according to these reactions. He found these diagnoses were more effective than those based on clinical examination. It is the total and absolute focus on the mental state of the sufferer alone that makes Dr. Bach's approach to health so exceptional. He believed that bringing balance to the mental and emotional state of a patient allowed the body to begin its healing process.

Flower power for emotional health

Dr. Bach formulated his flower essences by preparing mother tinctures from plant material and natural spring water, using either the sun or boiling method. He then mixed the tincture with a portion of grape alcohol, which acted as a preservative. He began to prescribe his wild flower essences according to the personality of his patients with immediate and remarkable results.[1] Today, Dr. Bach's gentle essences are used all over the world by individuals, medical and other healthcare practitioners, massage therapists, dentists, veterinarians and counselors.

I have personally used *Rescue Remedy,* the most popular of all the formulas. I truly believe that God has provided everything we need in creation for the balance of our body, mind and spirit. I consider these flower essences to be another one of His many gifts to us to be used to bring relief in times of emotional distress. These essences do not, however, replace the need for a life of faith and prayer that reflects our trust in God, especially when we are in emotional turmoil. Of course, this fact applies to all natural and medical remedies.

How the flower essences work

You are probably wondering what the Bach Flower Essences really are. There are thirty-eight essences, homeopathically prepared from the flowers of nonpoisonous plants, bushes and trees. Each is intended to treat a specific mental and emotional state of the patient. These natural formulas aim to relieve the effects that negative emotions or attitudes have on the mind and body, which then allows the body's own physical system to fight disease and the associated stress.

You will be pleased to know that the Bach Flower Essences are safe and natural, have no side effects and will not interfere with any other form of treatment, including nutritional, herbal and prescription medication. What's more, you do not have to be physically ill to benefit from the essences. In times of emotional difficulty, they can help restore balance before any physical symptoms appear. The following questionnaire and guide to discovering your own personal formula is reprinted by permission of Nelson Bach, USA, LTD. Bach Flower Essences can be purchased at most health food stores, by calling 1-800-314-BACH or at www.NelsonBach.com.

HOW TO TAKE BACH FLOWER ESSENCES

These healing essences can be prepared in two different ways. You can simply add two drops of the chosen essences to a glass of water or juice and sip it throughout the day. Or you can place two drops of each essence into a 1-ounce amber glass dropper bottle filled three-quarters with spring water, combining up to six or seven essences in your dosage bottle. You may want to add a teaspoon of brandy, apple cider vinegar or vegetable glycerin as a preservative. This is your treatment bottle.

You would take four drops by mouth a minimum of four times per day, particularly upon rising in the morning and before bedtime. (If you choose Rescue Remedy as part of your formula, it would be considered one essence and you would use four drops.)

For those unable to swallow or who are alcohol sensitive, these essences can be applied externally by moistening the lips, wrists and temples.

Guide to your personal formula

When you first begin reading the descriptions of the type of people for which each essence is prescribed, it may seem as if they all apply to you. However, you should try to limit your combination to a maximum of six or seven essences. As you read the questions under each essence, check the box to answer *yes* to any question you feel strongly applies to you at this moment. If you answer *yes* to all questions in any one group, that particular essence should be a part of your formula.

DISCOVERING YOUR ESSENCES

FOR THOSE WHO...	INDICATOR QUESTIONS	ESSENCE
Hide worries behind a brave face; are distressed by arguments, quarrels and confrontation; often turn to alcohol, drugs or comfort eating to help cope	❏ Do you find yourself hiding your worries behind a cheerful, smiling face in an attempt to conceal your pain from others? ❏ Are you distressed by arguments and quarrels, often "giving in " to avoid any conflict? ❏ When you feel life's pressures weighing you down, do you often turn to drugs, alcohol, or other outside influences to help you cope?	*Agrimony*
Experience apprehension for no known reason; are seized by sudden fears and anxieties; have feelings of unexplained anxious foreboding, dread.	❏ Do you have feelings of apprehension or uneasiness with no known cause? ❏ Do you worry that something bad may happen, but you're not sure what? ❏ Do you awaken with a sense of fear and anxiety of what the day will bring?	*Aspen*
Are critical and intolerant of others, unable and unwilling to make allowances; are convinced that they are right and everyone else is wrong; are perfectionists to the extreme.	❏ Do the habits and shortcomings of others annoy you? ❏ Do you find yourself being overly critical and intolerant, usually looking for what someone has done wrong and not right? ❏ Do you prefer to work or be alone because the seeming foolishness of others irritates you?	*Beech*

DISCOVERING YOUR ESSENCES

FOR THOSE WHO...	INDICATOR QUESTIONS	ESSENCE
Are weak willed, easily exploited or imposed upon; usually timid, quiet and passive; act out of subservience rather than a spirit of willing cooperation.	❑ Are you unable to say *no* to those who constantly impose upon your good nature? ❑ Do you tend to be timid and shy, easily influenced by those stronger in nature than yourself? ❑ Do you often deny your own needs in order to please others?	*Centaury*
Doubt their own judgment and seek confirmation of others; may be wise, educated and intuitive, yet constantly seek and follow the advice of others rather than trusting themselves.	❑ Do you constantly question your own decisions and judgment? ❑ Are you often seeking advice and confirmation from other people, mistrusting your own wisdom? ❑ Do you change direction often, first going one way, then another because you lack the confidence in yourself to stick with one direction?	*Cerato*
Experience uncontrolled, irrational thoughts; fear they may explode and give way to violent impulses and fits of rage. NOTE: If symptoms are severe, help from a good therapist is recommended.	❑ Do you fear losing control of yourself? ❑ Are you afraid of hurting yourself or others? ❑ Do you have a tendency to act irrationally and violently, exploding into unexplained fits of rage and anger?	*Cherry Plum*
Refuse to learn by experience and continually repeat the same mistakes; do their best to forget past difficulties and thus have no solid basis on which to base future decisions.	❑ Do you find yourself making the same mistakes over and over again such as choosing the wrong type of partner or staying in a job you dislike? ❑ Do you fail to learn from your experiences? ❑ Does it take you longer to advance in life because you are slow to learn from past mistakes?	*Chestnut Bud*

DISCOVERING YOUR ESSENCES

FOR THOSE WHO...	INDICATOR QUESTIONS	ESSENCE
Are overpossessive (self-centered), clinging and overprotective, especially of loved ones; expect others to conform to their values and are critical and argumentative when they do not; are interfering, talkative, self-pitying and easily offended.	❏ Are you possessive and manipulative of those you care for? ❏ Do you need to be needed? ❏ Do you feel unloved and unappreciated by your loved ones "after all you've done for them"?	*Chicory*
Are inattentive, dreamy, absent-minded and practicing mental escapism; like to be alone and avoid confrontation by withdrawing; show lack of interest.	❏ Do you often feel spacey and out of touch with the "real world"? ❏ Do you find yourself preoccupied and dreamy, unable to concentrate for any length of time? ❏ Are you drowsy and listless, sleeping more often then necessary?	*Clematis*
Are filled with self-disgust and detestation; are ashamed of ailments; have "symptoms" like obsessive house cleaning, frequent hand washing or obsession with trivialities.	❏ Are you obsessed with cleanliness? ❏ Are you embarrassed and ashamed of yourself physically, finding yourself unattractive? ❏ Do you tend to concentrate on small physical conditions such as pimples or marks, neglecting more serious problems?	*Crab Apple*
Are overwhelmed by responsibility; take on too much work while neglecting experience temporary depression, exhaustion and loss of self-esteem.	❏ Are you often overwhelmed by your responsibilities? ❏ Do you feel inadequate when it comes to dealing with the tasks ahead of you? ❏ Do you become depressed and exhausted when faced with your everyday commitments?	*Elm*

DISCOVERING YOUR ESSENCES

FOR THOSE WHO...	INDICATOR QUESTIONS	ESSENCE
Suffer from despondency; become easily depressed and discouraged when things go wrong or difficulties arise; are easily disheartened by small setbacks	❑ Do you become discouraged and depressed when things go wrong? ❑ Are you easily disheartened when faced with difficult situations? ❑ Does your pessimistic attitude prevent you from making an effort to accomplish something?	*Gentian*
Pessimistic, defeatist and "oh, what's the use!"; very often are suffering from chronic illness and have been told (or have come to believe) that nothing can be done for them; have no faith the treatments they are undergoing will work.	❑ Do you feel despondent and hopeless, at the end of your rope both mentally and physically? ❑ Do you lack confidence that things will get better in your life and therefore make no effort to improve your circumstances? ❑ Do you believe that nothing can be done to relieve your pain and suffering?	*Gorse*
Are talkative, obsessed with their own troubles and experiences; need an audience and dislike being alone; fail to realize they are often avoided because they sap other people's vitality.	❑ Are you totally self-absorbed, concerned only about yourself and your own problems and ailments? ❑ Do you talk incessantly, not interested in what anyone else has to say? ❑ Do you dislike being alone, always seeking the companionship of others?	*Heather*
Are filled with hatred, envy, jealousy and suspicions; unconsciously suffer from insecurity, yet project aggression to the world at large; lack the ability to feel love.	❑ Are you full of jealousy and hate? ❑ Do you mistrust others' intentions, feeling that people have "ulterior motives"? ❑ Do you feel great anger toward other people?	*Holly*

DISCOVERING YOUR ESSENCES

FOR THOSE WHO...	INDICATOR QUESTIONS	ESSENCE
Live in the past and are nostalgic, homesick; lack the ability to change the present because of constantly looking at the past, usually out of fear.	❑ Do you find yourself living in the past, nostalgic and homesick for the "way it was"? ❑ Are you unable to change present circumstances because you look back, never forward? ❑ Are you dissatisfied with your accomplishments?	*Honeysuckle*
Suffer the "Monday morning" feeling of procrastination; find it difficult to face everyday problems and responsibilities in spite of the fact that they manage to get things done.	❑ Do you often feel too tired to face the day ahead? ❑ Do you feel overworked or bored with your life? ❑ Do you lack enthusiasm and therefore tend to procrastinate?	*Hornbeam*
Are impatient and irritable; act, think and speak quickly but are frustrated and irritated by slow coworkers, so often they wind up working alone.	❑ Are you impatient and irritable with others who seem to do things too slowly for you? ❑ Do you prefer to work alone? ❑ Do you feel a sense of urgency in everything you do, always rushing to get through things?	*Impatiens*
Lack self-confidence; feel inferior; fear failure; won't try for fear of failing.	❑ Do you lack self-confidence? ❑ Do you feel inferior and often become discouraged? ❑ Are you so sure that you will fail and therefore do not even attempt things?	*Larch*
Suffer a fear of known things; are characterized by shyness and timidity; fear accidents, pain, poverty, public speaking, unemployment, etc. and are unable to speak about their fears.	❑ Do you have fears of known things, i.e., illness, death, pain, heights, darkness, the dentist, etc.? ❑ Are you shy, overly sensitive and often afraid? ❑ When you are confronted with a frightening situation, do you become too paralyzed to act?	*Mimulus*

DISCOVERING YOUR ESSENCES

FOR THOSE WHO...	INDICATOR QUESTIONS	ESSENCE
Describe a "dark cloud" that descends, making one saddened and low for no known reason; are truly exposed to the deepest gloom.	❑ Do you feel deep gloom, which seems to quickly descend for no apparent reason and lifts just as suddenly? ❑ Do you feel your moods swinging back and forth? ❑ Do you feel depressed without knowing why?	*Mustard*
Are normally strong and courageous, but no longer able to struggle bravely against illness and/or adversity; are overachievers with a strong sense of duty; hide their tiredness because they are afraid to appear weak in front of others.	❑ Are you exhausted but feel the need to struggle on against all odds? ❑ Do you have a strong sense of duty and dependability, carrying on no matter what obstacles stand in your way? ❑ Do you neglect your own needs in order to complete a task?	*Oak*
Are fatigued, drained of energy; suffer the type of exhaustion that sets in after a prolonged period of strain; everything becomes a monumental effort; live a life lacking zest.	❑ Do you feel utterly and completely exhausted? ❑ Are you totally drained of all energy with no reserves left, finding it difficult to carry on? ❑ Is everything an effort? Does your life lack zest?	*Olive*
Have a guilt complex; blame self even for mistakes of others; are always apologizing; feel undeserving and unworthy, which in turn destroys the joy of living.	❑ Are you full of guilt and self-reproach? ❑ Do you blame yourself for everything that goes wrong, including the mistakes of others? ❑ Do you set overly high standards for yourself, never satisfied with your achievements?	*Pine*
Are obsessed by care and concern for others; constantly fear the worst; live in dreaded anticipation of some nonspecific but definitely unfortunate thing happening to their loved ones.	❑ Are you excessively concerned and worried for your loved ones? ❑ Do you constantly worry that harm may come to those you care for? ❑ Are you distressed and disturbed by other people's problems?	*Red Chestnut*

DISCOVERING YOUR ESSENCES

FOR THOSE WHO...	INDICATOR QUESTIONS	ESSENCE
Become suddenly alarmed, scared or panicky, which often occurs after being in an accident or narrowly avoiding or witnessing an accident; feel frozen and helpless with fear due to an acute threat, sickness, natural disaster, etc.	❏ Do you feel terror and panic? ❏ Do you become helpless and frozen in the face of your fear? ❏ Do you suffer from nightmares?	*Rock Rose*
Are rigid minded and self-denying; are opinionated and dogmatic; are self-dominating to the point of self-martyrdom; are much too self-concerned to interfere in or connect with other people's lives.	❏ Are you inflexible in your approach to life, always striving for perfection? ❏ Are you so rigid in your ideals that you deny yourself the simple pleasures of life? ❏ Are you overly concerned with diet, exercise, work and spiritual disciplines?	*Rock Water*
Are filled with uncertainty, indecision, vacillation and fluctuating moods; waste time and miss opportunities because their up-and-down mood swings make them unreliable.	❏ Do you find it difficult to decide when faced with a choice of two possibilities? ❏ Do you lack concentration? Are you always fidgety and nervous? ❏ Do your moods change from one extreme to another: joy to sadness, optimism to pessimism, laughing to crying?	*Scleranthus*
Suffer serious distress and unhappiness under adverse conditions, all the effects of serious news, fright following an accident, etc.	❏ Have you suffered a shock in your life such as an accident, loss of a loved one, terrible news or illness? ❏ Are you numbed or withdrawn as a result of recent traumatic events in your life? ❏ Have you suffered a loss or grief from which you have never recovered?	*Star of Bethlehem*

DISCOVERING YOUR ESSENCES

FOR THOSE WHO...	INDICATOR QUESTIONS	ESSENCE
Suffer utter dejection and a bleak outlook; experience anguish so great it seems unbearable and all endurance seems gone.	❏ Do you suffer from extreme mental anguish? ❏ Do you feel that you have reached the limits of what you could possibly endure? ❏ Do you feel as though the future holds nothing for you?	*Sweet Chestnut*
Overenthusiastic with fanatical beliefs; strong-willed with strong views, especially about what they consider to be injustice; often so enthusiastic that they alienate potential allies.	❏ Do you feel tense and high strung? ❏ Do you have strong opinions, and only yours are the right ones? ❏ Is your overenthusiasm almost to the point of being fanatical?	*Vervain*
Are dominating, inflexible, tyrannical, autocratic and arrogant; are capable, gifted and ambitious and use their abilities to bully others; are proud and usually ruthlessly greedy for power.	❏ Do you tend to be domineering and overbearing? ❏ Do you feel the need to always be right? ❏ Are you inflexible and feel you know more than anyone else?	*Vine*
Need assistance in adjustment to transition or change, e.g. puberty, menopause, divorce or new surroundings; have definite ideas but who are occasionally diverted by the strong opinions of others.	❏ Are you experiencing any change in your life—a move, new job, loss of someone loved, new relationship, divorce, puberty, menopause, giving up an addiction? ❏ Are you distracted by outside influences? ❏ Do you need to make a break from strong forces or attachments in your life that may be holding you back?	*Walnut*

DISCOVERING YOUR ESSENCES

FOR THOSE WHO...	INDICATOR QUESTIONS	ESSENCE
Are proud, reserved and enjoy being alone; though often gentle and self-reliant, nevertheless can exude a sense of superiority that makes them appear aloof and condescending.	❑ Do you appear to others to be aloof and overly proud? ❑ Do you have a tendency to be withdrawn and prefer to be alone when faced with too many external distractions? ❑ Do you bear your grief and sorrow in silence?	*Water Violet*
Suffer persistent unwanted thoughts; are preoccupied with some worry or episode; have mental arguments that go around and around and lead to a troubled, depressed mind.	❑ Do you find your head full of persistent, unwanted thoughts that prevent concentration? ❑ Do you relive unhappy events or arguments over and over again? ❑ Are you unable to sleep at times because your mind seems to be cluttered with mental arguments that go round and round?	*White Chestnut*
Have ambition and talents but waste those gifts through a lack of direction; are frustrated because they are aware that life is passing them by; need help to determine their intended path in life.	❑ Do you find yourself in a complete state of uncertainty over major life decisions? ❑ Are you displeased with your lifestyle and feel dissatisfied with your achievements? ❑ Do you have ambition but feel that life is passing you by?	*Wild Oat*
Face life with resignation and apathy; do not complain, but simply plod unhappily on whether facing illness, a monotonous life or poor working conditions; miss even the simplest of life's pleasures because their apathetic behavior assures that their condition will not change.	❑ Are you apathetic and resigned to whatever may happen in your life? ❑ Do you have the attitude, "I will just live with it"? ❑ Do you lack the motivation to improve the quality of your life?	*Wild Rose*

| Are filled with resentment, bitterness and "poor old me!"; start to begrudge other people's good fortune; are grumbling and irritable, enjoying spreading gloom. | ❏ Do you feel resentful and bitter?
 ❏ Do you have difficulty forgiving and forgetting?
 ❏ Do you feel life is unfair and find yourself taking less and less interest in the things you used to enjoy? | *Willow* |

Rescue Remedy

For people who find themselves in emergency stress situations, Rescue Remedy is the only *combination* of essences (Cherry Plum, Clematis, Impatiens, Rock Rose, Star of Bethlehem) formulated and recognized by Dr. Bach himself. Rescue Remedy will comfort, reassure and calm those who have received serious news, severe upset or startling experiences that result in falling into a numbed, bemused state of mind.

Rescue Remedy can be used as well just before bed to calm a troubled mind or before any stressful situation such as exams, doctor or dentist appointments and public speaking. Rescue Remedy also comes in cream form that can be used topically on burns, stings and sprains or even as a massage cream.

AROMATHERAPY

Aromatherapy is a safe, pleasant way to lift your mood and relieve stress. Smell is the most rapid of your five senses. The aroma of essential oil molecules works through hormone-like chemicals to produce healing results. Scents and odors influence the hypothalamus and other glands responsible for hormone levels, metabolism and insulin. These glands monitor stress levels, appetite, body temperature and even sex drive. When you smell an aroma, that sensual information is directly relayed to the hypothalamus (part of a large gland that lies underneath your breastbone), where your motivations, moods, emotions and creativity all begin. Different aromas evoke different responses as they influence your glandular functions.

Actual studies of brain waves show that scents like lavender increase alpha brain waves, which are associated with relaxation, while scents like jasmine boost beta waves, which are linked to alertness. Aromatherapy works by stimulating a release of neurotransmitters once an essential oil is inhaled. Neurotransmitters are brain chemicals responsible for pain reduction and pleasant feelings. This is a brief scientific explanation of how aromatherapy calms, sedates and uplifts the body, mind and spirit.

Stop and smell the roses

Ever wonder where the proverbs of our forefathers came from? Whether or not they understood the science of what they were saying, they knew that stopping to smell the roses was a very wise thing to do. The effects of aromatherapy are immediate and profound on the central nervous system. Essential oils are most commonly used to counteract stress, which affects the mind and emotions. In addition, aromatherapy gives a sense of well-being by releasing mood-inducing neurochemicals in the brain. Aromatherapy promotes relaxation, alertness, restful sleep and physical relaxation. It can also increase energy.

Aromatherapy has been proven beneficial in helping to prevent panic attacks. I personally can attest to this. You'll be pleased to know, as we have mentioned, that stress reduction is an aromatherapy specialty. Listed below are essential oils that will help your body, mind and spirit as you continue on your journey to total wellness. They are a wonderful healing tool.

CHOOSE YOUR AROMATHERAPY

FOR STRESS

- Lavender: Balances your nerves and emotions. It calms the heart and helps to lower high blood pressure.

- Sandalwood: Good for sleep and relaxation.

- Clary Sage: Promotes feelings of well-being, calms nerves, lifts the mood and diminishes stress.

FOR DEPRESSION

- Jasmine: Very good for depression because it is uplifting and soothing.

- Lemon: Uplifting.

- Neroli: Relieves depression, insomnia, stress and anxiety.

FOR MOTIVATION AND ENERGY

- Ginger: Quickens and sharpens the senses. Helps memory.

- Rosemary: Clears the brain and enhances memory.

- Peppermint: Energizes.

Because the strength of essential oils is very concentrated, they should be mixed with a "carrier oil" such as almond oil in a ratio of fifteen drops of your aromatherapy essence to four ounces of oil. Just add a few drops of the essential oil and massage the body. You may also inhale them using a steam inhaler or a diffuser. Do not inhale them for more than fifteen minutes at a time. People with medical conditions such as blood pressure problems or asthma may have negative reactions to essential oils. Be sure to consult your healthcare professional if you have any doubts about how your condition will respond.

BATH ESSENTIALS

Do you want an attitude change or a little more energy? Try a different aromatherapy bath each night of the week, and you'll be surprised at your fresh outlook on life. Some essences are stronger than others and are used for different effects, so count out just a few drops of some common scents and get revitalized. If you are just beginning aromatherapy, I recommend you choose one or two of the following essential oils to put in your bath:

Restful bath

For maximum relaxation, I suggest you add to a tubful of water one of these essential oils: chamomile (two drops), cypress (five drops), orange blossom (two drops) or lavender (six drops).

No-more-blahs bath

Try lemon (four drops), peppermint (four drops), basil (three drops) or bergamot (three drops).

Spicy bath

Feel fresh with geranium (three drops), lavender (six drops), juniper (five drops) or cardamom (four drops).

Wake-up bath

For a stimulating bath, use basil (three drops), peppermint (four drops), juniper (five drops), hyssop (three drops) or rosemary (five drops).

Tension bath

Ease your way through the end of the week with bergamot (three drops), geranium (three drops) or lavender (six drops).

A growing number of medical doctors believe that if natural products like flower essences and aromatherapy oils were used, medical risks and side effects of more invasive or chemical (drug) therapies would be considerably lessened. It is a simple choice to make to see if your condition responds to these powerful natural therapies that many people have found helpful to their health.

Part Two

Determine Your Personal Health Needs

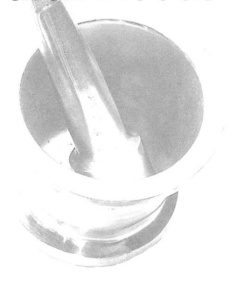

BALANCING THE FIVE SYSTEMS OF THE BODY

Natural medicine, as we have discussed, focuses on whole-body health. By balancing the five key systems of the body—gastrointestinal, endocrine, structural neurological, immune and visceral—optimal health can be achieved. In this section you will find system questionnaires for each of the five systems of your body. These questionnaires were developed by Sylvia Kreutle, M.S., founder of HealthQuest, Inc.[1] (See www.hquest.com for more information.) Check the areas of symptomatic difficulty you are presently experiencing. Use this information as your indicator in terms of what system of your body you need to focus your attention to improve your health.

Several checks in any given area or section will alert you to focus your attention on that particular body system. Remember, when one system is out of balance, it affects the other four systems. Like a lame horse in a team of horses that cannot pull its weight and therefore taxes the other horses, so when one body system is weak or cannot pull its weight, the other systems have to pick up the slack and thus become overtaxed. Balance is key.

After taking the five screenings, refer to the Systems Analysis Guide to see where your imbalances or weaknesses are. Then use the A-to-Z health-building section to address the root of your problem so that you can move toward optimal health.

It is imperative that you take inventory of your body in this way to see just where your weaknesses are. You may find that some of your complaints seem to run in your family or are hereditary. Don't let this alarm you. Remember, "to be forewarned is to be forearmed." This simply means that those weak areas need more attention or strengthening.

While working to overcome my personal health struggles, my studies took me on a journey through all avenues of alternative medicine. I found that in Chinese medicine it is believed that if you have moved into chronic illness of any kind, a balancing principle must be applied. That means balancing all five systems of our bodies: gastrointestinal, endocrine, structural neurological, immune and visceral.

This balancing of the body's systems is known as the principle of regeneration. Regeneration differs from medicine because it has nothing at all to do with treating disease. To treat a disease, medicine first names it, then seeks a specific cure for it. The regeneration principle, in contrast, holds that there are no specific diseases, only internal weaknesses, usually reversible, that manifest in certain symptom patterns. By using the symptom pattern to discern the weakness and then strengthening the body system, we create optimal conditions that allow the symptoms to go away, replaced by the vitality and balance of health.

This regeneration principle was a blessing to my physical body. We must discover and live principles of healthful living that will restore balance to the immune system. The Bible declares:

> My people are destroyed for lack of knowledge.
>
> —Hosea 4:6, KJV

Keep firmly in mind that as you employ the powerful remedies of natural medicine you must shift your thinking from the disease-oriented point of view that seeks an external cure to a specific disease, to embrace the regeneration principle that seeks to strengthen and balance your body. From this perspective, symptoms are regarded only as signs of possible weakness.

Vitamins, medicines, herbs, potions, lotions and so forth heal nothing! God made our bodies with the innate ability to heal. These natural remedies help support the body, strengthen the weak areas and let the healing begin! Again, let me emphasize your need to work in partnership with your doctor. It is a winning combination.

GASTROINTESTINAL QUESTIONNAIRE

PART 1: DIGESTION

Section A
- ❑ Abdomen bloats after eating
- ❑ Loss of taste for meat
- ❑ Excessive upper or lower abdominal gas 2–3 hours after eating
- ❑ Belching or burping after meals
- ❑ Frequent upset stomach
- ❑ Known food allergies
- ❑ Fasting affects your stomach
- ❑ Coated tongue
- ❑ Treated for anemia many times without success
- ❑ Frequent constipation and/or diarrhea
- ❑ Told you have a B_{12} or folic acid deficiency
- ❑ Frequent heartburn
- ❑ Vomiting of undigested food
- ❑ Indigestion 2–3 hours after eating

Section B
- ❑ Chronic burning sensation in the stomach
- ❑ Stomach pains just before meals
- ❑ Stomach pains relieved by drinking milk/cream
- ❑ Take antacids frequently
- ❑ Stomach complaints aggravated by worry or tension
- ❑ Frequent meals relieve your stomach pains
- ❑ Diagnosed with an ulcer
- ❑ Experience sudden, acute indigestion
- ❑ Pains subside when vacationing or relaxed
- ❑ History of gastritis or ulcers
- ❑ Stool is black when you are not taking an iron supplement
- ❑ Acute stomach pain after eating or lying down
- ❑ Spicy food or caffeine causes diarrhea
- ❑ Excessive use of aspirin and other anti-inflammatory medications (including steroids)

Section C
- ❑ Lower bowel gas several hours after eating
- ❑ Bloating after meals
- ❑ Stools are shiny and/or poorly formed
- ❑ Difficult to gain weight
- ❑ Skin is dry and flaky
- ❑ Experience diarrhea frequently
- ❑ Fiber irritates your diarrhea
- ❑ Hair is brittle and dry
- ❑ Alternate between diarrhea and constipation
- ❑ Known food allergies
- ❑ Frequent stomach cramps
- ❑ Mucus in your stools

GASTROINTESTINAL QUESTIONNAIRE (CONTINUED)

❑ Pain on inside of left shoulder blade
❑ Pain on left side of abdomen (lower rib cage)
❑ Pass large amounts of foul-smelling stool
❑ Fibrous foods and roughage cause constipation
❑ Problems with acne
❑ Low self-esteem

Section D
❑ Chemical sensitivities
❑ Exposure to toxic chemicals/drugs/alcohol
❑ Fatigue
❑ Frequent belching/burping
❑ Yellow in the whites of your eyes
❑ Constipation
❑ Abdominal cramps
❑ Stools are light-colored and foul smelling
❑ Consistent bloating and gas
❑ Bad breath (halitosis) and/or body odor
❑ Eye problems
❑ Dry skin or hair
❑ Bitter, metallic taste in mouth in mornings
❑ Painful bowel movements
❑ Skin on your feet peels
❑ Pain at right shoulder blade
❑ Pain radiates down outside of your legs
❑ Pain on the right side of your abdomen
❑ Frequent bad dreams/nightmares
❑ Fatty foods cause nausea and distress
❑ Chronic anger, frustration and/or irritability
❑ Wake regularly between 1 and 3 A.M.
❑ Red blood present in your stool
❑ Triglyceride level above 115
❑ Cholesterol level above 200
❑ High LDL, low HDL cholesterol
❑ Diagnosed with hepatitis/jaundice
❑ History of gallbladder attacks or gallstones

PART 2: ELIMINATION

Section A
❑ Frequent diarrhea with no apparent cause
❑ Bowel movements thin and pencil-like
❑ History of constipation
❑ Painful bowel movements
❑ Alternating constipation and diarrhea
❑ Blood in your stool
❑ Mucus in your stool
❑ History of antibiotic use

GASTROINTESTINAL QUESTIONNAIRE (CONTINUED)

❑ History of vaginal yeast infections
❑ Abdominal pain and tenderness
❑ Excess gas and flatulence
❑ Suffer from anxiety or depression
❑ Frequently sick with a cold or infection

Section B
❑ Do you have hemorrhoids?
❑ Do you have itching, burning pain and/or inflammation in the rectal area?
❑ Do you have bright red blood on the tissue paper after a bowel movement?

VISCERAL QUESTIONNAIRE

PART 1: CARDIOVASCULAR

Section A
❑ Chest pain radiating to left arm and/or left neck
❑ Frequent leg cramps
❑ Dizziness
❑ Heartburn
❑ Breathing difficulties
❑ Minor exercise causes exhaustion
❑ Feel anxious or uptight frequently
❑ Feet and ankles swell
❑ Heart sometimes "flip-flops" in chest
❑ Hacking cough
❑ Diagonal crease in earlobe
❑ High blood pressure
❑ Rapid heartbeat (more than 90 beats/minute)
❑ Diagnosed with a heart condition

Section B
❑ Extremities often "fall asleep"
❑ Fingers and toes are often cold
❑ Ankles swell during the afternoon
❑ Out of breath after slight exertion
❑ Difficult to breathe when lying down
❑ Numbness/heaviness in arms and/or legs
❑ Nose and/or face have tiny "spider veins"
❑ Frequent tingling sensation in legs/fingers
❑ Frequent cramps in legs when walking
❑ Difficulty concentrating
❑ Frequent headaches
❑ Frequent ringing in your ears

VISCERAL QUESTIONNAIRE (CONTINUED)

Section C
- ❏ Diagnosed with high blood pressure (greater than 140/90 mm/Hg)
- ❏ Frequent headaches
- ❏ Dizziness
- ❏ Fatigued often
- ❏ Difficulty breathing
- ❏ Insomnia
- ❏ Suffer from restlessness or emotional instability
- ❏ Intestinal complaints

PART 2: RESPIRATORY

Section A
- ❏ Chronic cough
- ❏ Breathing difficulties
- ❏ Chest pains
- ❏ Wheezing
- ❏ Diagnosed with asthma
- ❏ History of bronchitis
- ❏ Recurrent sinus infections
- ❏ Hypersensitive to environmental pollutants
- ❏ Excessive mucus in throat and nose
- ❏ Frequent sore throats
- ❏ Work around chemicals/pollutants/radiation
- ❏ Chronic pain around rib cage
- ❏ Smoker
- ❏ Coughing up blood

PART 3: GENITO-URINARY

Section A
- ❏ Burning and pain on urination
- ❏ Increased urinary frequency and urgency
- ❏ Lower abdominal pain
- ❏ Recurrent bladder infections
- ❏ Tend to pass urine when you cough or sneeze
- ❏ Urinary incontinence (can't hold urine)
- ❏ Wake up frequently at night to urinate
- ❏ Tendency to drip after urinating
- ❏ Foul-smelling or dark urine
- ❏ History of bladder infections
- ❏ History of antibiotic use for bladder infections

Section B
- ❏ Low- to mid-back pain (near lower rib cage)
- ❏ Cloudy urine
- ❏ Foul-smelling and/or strong-smelling urine
- ❏ Fever/chills
- ❏ Nausea/vomiting
- ❏ Fatigue around 4 P.M.

VISCERAL QUESTIONNAIRE (CONTINUED)

PART 4:
EYES AND EARS

❑ Ankle edema or pitting edema (skin of extremities)
❑ Unknown fears
❑ History of antibiotic use for urinary tract infections
❑ History of kidney infections
❑ Blood in urine

Section A: Eyes
❑ Experience any visual problems
❑ Night blindness
❑ Cloudy vision
❑ Discharge from your eyes
❑ Pain, swelling or redness of your eyes
❑ Diagnosed with any eye disorder (cataracts, glaucoma, macular degeneration, etc.)

Section B: Ears
❑ General ear pain
❑ Earache
❑ Red, swollen eardrum
❑ Dull, throbbing pain in ear
❑ Ringing in ears
❑ Static sounds in ears
❑ Current ear infection

ENDOCRINE QUESTIONNAIRE

PART 1:
GLANDULAR

Section A
❑ Get dizzy when you stand up quickly
❑ Lose your vision when you stand quickly
❑ Weak and shaky often
❑ Sensitive to bright light, sunlight or headlights
❑ Have allergies (hay fever, asthma, rashes, etc.)
❑ "Lump in throat" that hurts when upset
❑ Sensitive to environmental pollutants
❑ Headache when standing up
❑ Low blood pressure
❑ Crave salt
❑ Heavy stress causes complete exhaustion
❑ Easily startled or frightened
❑ Loud noises cause your heart to pound
❑ Form "goose bumps" easily
❑ Perfectionist
❑ Dark circles under your eyes
❑ Difficult time breathing

ENDOCRINE QUESTIONNAIRE (CONTINUED)

Section B

- ❏ Experience chronic fatigue
- ❏ Gain weight easily
- ❏ Sensitive to cold weather
- ❏ Easily depressed
- ❏ Slow heart rate
- ❏ Swollen eyes or face
- ❏ Chronic constipation
- ❏ Dry, flaky skin
- ❏ Easily irritated
- ❏ Slowed or slurred speech
- ❏ Excess hair loss
- ❏ Hair and/or nails are brittle and dry
- ❏ Recurrent infections
- ❏ Allergic reactions
- ❏ Headaches
- ❏ Heavy menstrual flow
- ❏ Suffer from PMS
- ❏ Painful periods
- ❏ Low sex drive
- ❏ Difficulty concentrating or remembering
- ❏ Cry easily
- ❏ Difficulty sleeping
- ❏ Cold hands and feet
- ❏ Ancillary temperature below 97.5°F

Section C

- ❏ Rapid heartbeat (more than 90 beats/minute)
- ❏ Bulging, swollen eyes
- ❏ Sweat excessively with moist skin and palms
- ❏ Increased appetite
- ❏ Chest pains
- ❏ Gastrointestinal disturbances
- ❏ Difficult to relax
- ❏ Insomnia
- ❏ Menstrual problems
- ❏ Rash or swelling in front of lower leg
- ❏ Diarrhea
- ❏ Enlarged thyroid (goiter)
- ❏ Experience tremors (trembling)
- ❏ Increased body temperature
- ❏ Fatigue
- ❏ Anxious and nervous
- ❏ Low tolerance to heat
- ❏ Lose weight easily

ENDOCRINE QUESTIONNAIRE (CONTINUED)

Section D
❑ Feel better after eating
❑ Fatigued if meal is missed
❑ Hungry for sweets
❑ Symptoms occur in afternoon or several hours after eating
❑ Memory problems and/or poor concentration
❑ Wake up at night feeling hungry
❑ Digestive complaints
❑ Headaches relieved by sweets or alcohol
❑ Anxiety/nervousness
❑ Rapid heart rate
❑ Extreme hunger
❑ Weak/shaky/jittery
❑ Irritable if meal is missed
❑ Dizzy when standing too quickly
❑ Double vision

Section E
❑ Irritable
❑ Frequent urination
❑ Weakness or fatigue
❑ Unusual hunger
❑ Excessive thirst
❑ Nausea/vomiting
❑ Cuts that will not heal
❑ Vision problems
❑ History of diabetes in your family
❑ Overweight
❑ Tingling/numbness in feet
❑ Skin infections/leg sores

Section F
❑ Abdominal bloating
❑ Redness and bloating of face
❑ Fatigue
❑ Overweight at the hips/waist (pear-shaped)
❑ Menstrual irregularities
❑ Lack of menstruation in younger girls
❑ Water retention/edema
❑ Thyroid problems
❑ Slowed growth in children
❑ Cold hands and feet
❑ Cold all over
❑ Infertility
❑ Sex drive reduced or lacking
❑ Chronic headaches at level of eyes

Endocrine Questionnaire (continued)

❏ Mental and/or emotional stress
❏ Abnormal thirst
❏ Excessive urination

Section G
❏ Very susceptible to infections
❏ Chronic swollen glands in neck/groin/armpit
❏ Frequent flu-like symptoms
❏ Irregular heartbeat
❏ Soreness in neck
❏ Infections last longer than seven days
❏ Over the age of fifty

Section H
❏ Lack of coordination in the dark
❏ Symptoms worse in the evening
❏ Difficulty waking in the morning
❏ Irregular sleep habits
❏ Symptoms worse in fall and/or winter

PART 2: FOR MALES ONLY

Section A
❏ Increased urinary frequency
❏ Need to urinate during the night
❏ Reduced urine flow with increased strain
❏ Difficulty in urinating or stopping urine flow
❏ Pain or burning during urination
❏ Discharge from penis after bowel movements
❏ Blood or pus in urine
❏ Back pain or leg pain
❏ Fever/chills
❏ Impotence (difficult to maintain an erection)
❏ Lost or diminished sex drive
❏ Prostate trouble

Section B
❏ Inability to achieve or maintain an erection
❏ Premature ejaculation
❏ Inability to ejaculate
❏ Low or diminished sex drive
❏ Currently taking medication (antihypertensives, tranquilizers or Tagamet)
❏ Inability to impregnate a woman
❏ Low sperm count

Section C
❏ Unusual discharge from penis
❏ Itchy genitals

ENDOCRINE QUESTIONNAIRE (CONTINUED)

❑ Swelling or pain in genital area
❑ Recent changes in urination (frequency, etc.)
❑ Burning in the genital area
❑ Bumps or blisters on the genitals
❑ Visible warts on genitals
❑ Diagnosed with sexually transmitted disease (herpes, gonorrhea, warts, etc.)

PART 2: FOR FEMALES ONLY

Section A
Do you have any of these symptoms during menstruation?
❑ Lower abdominal pain
❑ Backache
❑ Pinching/pain sensations in inner thighs
❑ Intense cramps right before period
❑ Abdominal bloating
❑ Sugar craving
❑ Light or heavy blood flow
❑ Anxious about getting your period
❑ Stay in bed the first few days of period
❑ Pain during period is getting worse

Section B
❑ Lack of menstruation
❑ Irregular periods
❑ Vaginal itching or abnormal discharge
❑ Low sex drive
❑ Regularly do strenuous exercise
❑ Fifteen years or older and haven't gotten your period
❑ Diagnosed or believe you have anorexia
❑ Unable to get pregnant
❑ 5–10 pounds under your ideal weight
❑ Have you had any miscarriages?
❑ Have you had any abortions?

Section C
Do you have any of these symptoms prior to menstruation?
❑ Depressed
❑ Altered sex drive
❑ Breast pain
❑ Backache
❑ Abdominal bloating
❑ Swelling in hands and feet
❑ Anxiety and/or suicidal feelings
❑ Easily irritated and/or mood swings
❑ Cramps
❑ Weight gain each month

ENDOCRINE QUESTIONNAIRE (CONTINUED)

❑ Crying for no apparent reason
❑ Sugar craving
❑ Headaches

Section D
❑ Small lumps in your breast
❑ Breast pain and tenderness
❑ Breast swelling/tender to touch
❑ Painful ovaries
❑ Lower abdominal pain
❑ History of breast cancer in your family
❑ Never been pregnant
❑ Recent Pap smear test positive
❑ Ovarian or uterine cysts
❑ Endometriosis
❑ Mother used D.E.S. (hormones) while pregnant with you
❑ Sudden onset of pain on one side of abdomen halfway between monthly cycles

Section E
❑ Hot flashes
❑ Weight gain
❑ Memory loss
❑ Irritability/mood swings
❑ Depression
❑ Vaginal dryness and pain
❑ Anxiety (sometimes followed by chills)
❑ Low sex drive/low arousal time
❑ Heart palpitations
❑ Water retention
❑ Night sweats and/or sweat throughout day
❑ Above symptoms and over age forty-five
❑ Have you had a hysterectomy?
❑ Diagnosed with osteoporosis

STRUCTURAL/NEUROLOGICAL QUESTIONNAIRE

PART 1: STRUCTURAL

Section A
❑ Experience muscle cramps
❑ Frequent muscle spasms
❑ Low back pain
❑ Leg muscles cramp at night
❑ Tight muscles
❑ Muscular discomfort or pain
❑ Muscle stiffness all over
❑ Muscle stiffness after a good night's sleep

Section B
❑ Mild early morning stiffness
❑ Loss or restriction of joint mobility
❑ Pain that is worse after using the joint
❑ Stiffness after periods of rest
❑ Creaking/cracking of joints
❑ Tenderness and swelling in certain areas
❑ Diagnosed with osteoarthritis
❑ Chronic fatigue and weakness
❑ Low-grade fever
❑ Joint stiffness and joint pain
❑ Painful, swollen joints
❑ Severe joint pain with inflammation
❑ Diagnosed with rheumatoid arthritis
❑ Severe pain in first joint of big toe
❑ Constipation/indigestion
❑ Headaches
❑ Heart or kidney problems
❑ Diagnosed with gout

Section C
❑ Have had spontaneous bone fractures
❑ Painful bones
❑ Eat red meat often
❑ Are you postmenopausal?
❑ Take anti-inflammatory medication often
❑ Smoker
❑ Drink alcohol excessively
❑ Taken synthetic thyroid medication for long period of time
❑ Have calcium deposits in joints
❑ Drink large amounts of soda and/of coffee
❑ Family history of osteoporosis
❑ Experienced early menopause (before forty-five years of age)
❑ Diagnosed with osteoporosis/osteomalacia
❑ Have a current bone fracture

STRUCTURAL/NEUROLOGICAL QUESTIONNAIRE (CONTINUED)

PART 2: NEUROLOGICAL

Section D
- ❏ Loss of range of joint motion
- ❏ Persistent back pain
- ❏ Localized joint pain or tenderness
- ❏ Swollen joints
- ❏ Prone to injury
- ❏ Double-jointed (over-flexible joints)
- ❏ Do you have tendonitis?
- ❏ Do you have bursitis?
- ❏ Do you have a slipped disc?
- ❏ Do you have a herniated disc?
- ❏ Are you recovering from a current injury?

Section A
- ❏ Experience tremors in hands and/or feet
- ❏ Often nervous or "on edge"
- ❏ Slurred speech
- ❏ Easily lose your balance
- ❏ Tire easily
- ❏ Easily irritated
- ❏ Frequent dizziness/lightheadedness
- ❏ Lack of coordination
- ❏ Memory problems
- ❏ Depression
- ❏ "Spaciness"
- ❏ Ringing in your ears
- ❏ Extremities numb easily
- ❏ Head and/or limbs feel heavy
- ❏ Blurred or double vision
- ❏ Convulsions
- ❏ Loss of muscle tone or muscle strength
- ❏ Diagnosed with shingles
- ❏ Lose temper easily, emotionally unsettled
- ❏ Hand tremors
- ❏ Hyperactive behavior

IMMUNE RESPONSE QUESTIONNAIRE

Section A
❑ Easily susceptible to infections
❑ Frequently catch a cold or flu
❑ Difficult to recuperate from a flu or cold
❑ Chronic swollen lymph glands
❑ Frequent sore throats
❑ Cuts or bruises heal slowly
❑ Hair grows slowly
❑ Frequent ear infections
❑ Cold sores or fever blisters
❑ Chronic low-grade fever
❑ Gums and/or nose bleeds easily
❑ Experience frequent runny nose
❑ Muscle aches and joint pain
❑ Frequently tired or fatigued, unrelieved by sleep

Section B
❑ Known chemical sensitivities
❑ Known environmental and/or food allergies
❑ Irritability/mood swings
❑ Frequent headaches and/or migraines
❑ Abnormal fatigue not helped by rest
❑ Postnasal drip
❑ Frequent sneezing attacks and/or hay fever
❑ Weight fluctuations of 4–5 pounds in one day accompanied by
   puffiness in face/ankles/fingers
❑ Chronic muscle aches and pains
❑ Suffer from asthma/breathing difficulties
❑ Eczema, hives or skin rashes
❑ Suffer from depression or crying spells
❑ Itchy eyes or nose
❑ Chronic runny nose
❑ Chronic stuffy nose
❑ Dark circles under eyes
❑ Frequent urination of bedwetting
❑ Swelling in joints
❑ Mouth or throat itches
❑ Chronic lymph gland swelling, especially in the throat area
❑ Acne
❑ Sweat for no apparent reason/hot flashes
❑ Suffer from irritable bowel, spastic colon or colitis
❑ Certain foods cause you to have a reaction (jitters, depression, ill
   feelings, etc.)
❑ Strong cravings for certain foods
❑ Pulse races after eating certain foods or for no apparent reason
❑ Mucus in stool

IMMUNE RESPONSE QUESTIONNAIRE (CONTINUED)

❑ Minor chronic complaints that always recur
❑ Feel best when you do not eat
❑ Hyperactive
❑ Abdominal pain after eating
❑ Alternating diarrhea and constipation

Section C
❑ Chronic fatigue, especially after eating
❑ Depression
❑ Recurrent digestive complaints
❑ Rectal itching
❑ Food and/or environmental allergies
❑ Severe PMS
❑ Feel "spacey"
❑ Poor memory
❑ Severe mood swings
❑ Anxiety/nervousness
❑ Recurrent fungal infections (athlete's foot, ringworm, "jock itch")
❑ Extreme chemical sensitivity
❑ Cannot tolerate perfumes or smoke
❑ Coated or sore tongue
❑ Prostatitis
❑ Recurrent vaginal or urinary infections
❑ Lightheadedness or feel drunk after minimal wine, beer or certain foods
❑ Respiratory problems
❑ Chronic skin rashes or acne
❑ Loss of libido/impotence
❑ Thrush (white fungus in mouth or vagina)
❑ Headaches/migraines
❑ Muscle and joint pains
❑ Low blood sugar
❑ History of frequent antibiotic use
❑ Taking or have taken birth control pills
❑ Crave sugar, breads or alcoholic beverages
❑ Endometriosis and/or infertility
❑ Above conditions get worse in moldy places like basements or damp climates
❑ Above conditions get worse after eating or drinking items that contain yeast or sugar

Section D
❑ Fatigue
❑ Depression
❑ Anxiety, nervousness and/or irritability
❑ High blood pressure

IMMUNE RESPONSE QUESTIONNAIRE (CONTINUED)

❑ Increased susceptibility to infections
❑ Headaches
❑ Digestive problems (colic, nausea, pain)
❑ Numbness/tingling/tremors
❑ Skin problems (rashes, eczema, psoriasis)
❑ Learning disabilities
❑ Ringing in your ears
❑ Muscle and joint pain
❑ Allergies/asthma
❑ Kidney and/or liver problems
❑ Constipation
❑ Memory problems
❑ Anemia
❑ Varied symptoms with no relief

Use this handy Systems Analysis Guide to determine which system of your body needs strengthening. The right column tells you the health-building section that will enable you to address your problem areas. Page numbers are also given at the first mention of the health-building section.

SYSTEMS ANALYSIS GUIDE

IMMUNE SYSTEM QUESTIONNAIRE

Section A	Basic Immune Function	Immune Health System (page 184)
Section B	Allergy (food or environmental)	Food Allergies (page 163)
Section C	Yeast/Fungal Involvement	Candidiasis (page 130)
Section D	Parasitic Involvement	Detoxification (page 21)

SYSTEMS ANALYSIS GUIDE

GASTROINTESTINAL SYSTEM QUESTIONNAIRE

DIGESTIVE FUNCTION

Section A	Hypo-acidity	Gastric Disease (page 166)
Section B	Hyperacidity	Gastric Disease
Section C	Pancreas/Small Intestine	Gastric Disease; Diabetes (page 151)
Section D	Liver/Gallbladder	Liver Problems (page 189); Gallbladder Disease (page 165)

ELIMINATION

Section A	Large Colon	Colon Health (page 139)
Section B	Capillary Fragility	Colon Health

SYSTEMS ANALYSIS GUIDE

STRUCTURAL/NEUROLOGICAL QUESTIONNAIRE

STRUCTURAL FUNCTION

Section A	Muscle Health	Arthritis (page 108); Sports Injuries (page 205)
Section B	Joint Health	Arthritis; Sports Injuries
Section C	Bone Health	Arthritis; Sports Injuries
Section D	Connective Tissue Health	Arthritis; Sports Injuries

NEUROLOGICAL FUNCTION

Section A	Neurological Health	Brain Drain (page 115)

SYSTEMS ANALYSIS GUIDE

VISCERAL SYSTEM QUESTIONNAIRE

CARDIOVASCULAR FUNCTION

Section A	Heart Health	Heart Attack and Related Heart Conditions (page 171)
Section B	Circulation	High Blood Pressure (Hypertension) (page 179)
Section C	Blood Pressure	High Blood Pressure (Hypertension)

RESPIRATORY FUNCTION

Section A	Lung Health	Asthma (page 111); Bronchitis (page 120)

GENITO-URINARY FUNCTION

Section A	Bladder Health	Bladder Infection (page 114)
Section B	Kidney Health	Kidney Problems (page 188)

EYES/EARS

Section A	Eye Health	Eye Health (page 159)
Section B	Ear Health	Earaches (page 155)

SYSTEMS ANALYSIS GUIDE

ENDOCRINE SYSTEM QUESTIONNAIRE

GLANDULAR HEALTH

Section A	Hypo-adrenia	Adrenal Exhaustion (page 92)
Section B	Low Thyroid/Hypothyroid	Hypothyroidism (page 182)
Section C	Hyperthyroid	Hypothyroidism
Section D	Hypoglycemia	Hypoglycemia (Low Blood Sugar) (page 181)
Section E	Hyperglycemia	Sugar Sabotage (page 26)
Section F	Pituitary Health	Stress (page 207)
Section G	Thymus Health	Immune System Health (page 184)
Section H	Pineal Health	Stress

Males Only

Section A	Prostate Health	Andropause (page 102)
Section B	Reproductive Health	Andropause
Section C	Genital Health	Andropause

Females Only

Section A	Dysmenorrhea (menstrual cramps)	PMS (page 195)
Section B	Amenorrhea	PMS
Section C	PMS	PMS
Section D	Fibrocystic Problems	Breast Disease (page 118)
Section F	Menopause/Hot Flashes	Menopause (page 192)

Part Three

———◆━✦━◆———

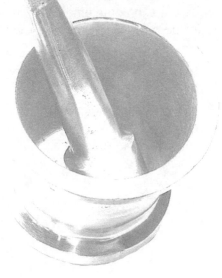

Family Health
Remedies
A-to-Z Ailment Guide

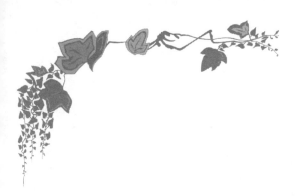

The material on the following pages will offer you natural healing options in a drugless format. Information regarding these ailments will include:

- ❦ Definition, most common symptoms and some causes of the ailment
- ❦ Dietary considerations
- ❦ Helpful medical treatments when appropriate
- ❦ Supplement support for the ailment
- ❦ Lifestyle choices to ease symptoms and support the healing process

Education is essential in your quest for vibrant health. That is the purpose of this family guide. Remember, alternative therapies should be pursued after consulting your healthcare provider. This guide is to be used as an educational reference tool only. I encourage you to have an ongoing dialogue with your healthcare professional. Always inform your doctor as to what vitamins and herbs you are taking, along with other natural therapies you are using.

Many physicians are open to natural medicine and have become more knowledgeable on how it can complement the protocol that they outline for their patients. It can be a beautiful marriage with one shared goal—*your health!*

Acne—Blemishes/Pimples

Acne is a condition that affects young and old alike. It can be a source of great shame and embarrassment and can hinder your social life, thereby leaving scars that are not only superficial but also deep within. There are many causes. The main one is pituitary gland and male hormone imbalance during the high growth years of adolescence and before menstruation. In addition, diet comes into play when it comes to acne outbreaks. A high-fat, fried-food, excessive-sugar diet sets the stage for this unwelcome condition. Heredity, poor liver function and poor elimination can also play a role in its development. In adulthood, some hormone therapies, allergies, cosmetics and, of course, the big one—STRESS—contribute to the occurrence of acne.

Definition
Acne is an inflammatory skin condition characterized by superficial skin eruptions that are caused by clogged skin pores.

Symptoms
Symptoms of acne include skin rash, whiteheads, blackheads, cysts, redness and scarring. It most commonly appears on the face, shoulders, trunk, arms and legs.

Dietary considerations
You will need to make some healthy choices regarding diet to allow your skin condition to heal. Eliminate white flour, sugar, chocolate, fried foods, fatty dairy foods, tobacco, tomatoes, peppers, eggplant and peanut butter, which are acne triggers. It will also be very healing to go on a three- to five-day juice cleansing fast during which you drink six glasses of water along with carrot, pineapple and papaya juices daily to clear out wastes.

Supplement support for acne
- Evening primrose oil: four to six capsules daily (essential fatty acids)
- Tea tree oil applied externally
- Digestive plant enzymes (especially pancreatin to digest oils) with meals
- Milk thistle extract (to detoxify liver for two to three months)
- Fresh pineapple (rub on face to reduce acne scars)
- A green drink daily (Kyo-Green by Wakunaga)
- Royal jelly
- Fiber for proper elimination
- Zinc: 30 mg morning and evening
- Vitamin C: 1000 mg morning and evening
- Acidophilus (especially if taking antibiotics)

In addition, you can try these natural healing approaches:

- Early morning sunlight on the face
- Daily exercise

- Plenty of rest
- Apple cider vinegar (dab on breakouts and sores daily)
- B-complex vitamin with extra pantothenic acid for stress-caused acne
- Stevia extract directly on breakouts

Medical treatment

There are various medical approaches to the treatment of acne that include use of antibiotics (tetracycline), synthetic vitamin A analogues, cortisone, chemical skin peels, dermabrasion and drainage of cysts.

Herbal cleanser

If you have trouble with boils, acne or other skin problems, use cleansing herbs or a detoxification program like Nature's Secret Ultimate Cleanse. This will help to cleanse your blood, liver and kidneys of toxic waste products. Acne is often the result of hormonal imbalance or toxicity of the blood or bowel.

Common questions from acne patients

Q. What causes blackheads?

A. Blackheads result when sebaceous oil combines with unreleased wastes that plug the pore.

Q. Why are whiteheads more dangerous?

A. Whiteheads have the potential for becoming inflamed and infected. Whiteheads happen when scales below the skin's surface become filled with sebaceous oil. They can spread under the skin and rupture and then spread the infection.

Q. What foods should I eat to help prevent an outbreak?

A. Eat plenty of fresh foods, whole grains, green vegetables, fish, brown rice, apples and low-fat dairy foods.

Q. What foods should I avoid?

A. White flour and sugar, candy, pies, pastries, caffeine, soda, fried foods and foods with a lot of preservatives. In other words—NO JUNK FOOD!

Q. How does a detoxification program help?

A. During detoxification with a good detox product, you can safely cleanse your blood, liver, colon and kidneys to rid your system of toxins that contribute not only to acne, but also to many of our modern-day degenerative diseases. A clean body will produce a clean complexion.

Q. I hate water. How important is it when it comes to getting rid of acne?

A. Very important. You want to keep the body flushed and properly hydrated each day to insure optimal functioning of every organ system. In addition, water helps speed up the detoxification process. I recommend six to eight glasses of bottled water daily.

Q. Is there anything "natural" that I can use to improve the appearance of my skin once acne has shown its ugly face?

A. Yes. God has provided wonderful remedies from nature. For acne scars, try rubbing fresh pineapple directly on the scars each day. Its enzyme activity from bromelain has been known to make a difference with consistent use. Also, try lemon juice or aloe vera gel before bed. Do not wash off. Rinse face in the morning. In addition, rub the affected areas with the inside of a papaya skin. Again, the enzyme papain will help to neutralize the acid wastes on the skin and help to heal the infected area. These remedies should be rotated and used on different days.

Q. I can't go without my makeup! What can I use?

A. Make sure to use water-based cosmetics only. Oil-based formulas are too clogging to already congested pores.

Q. I am always constipated. How does this factor in when it comes to acne?

A. If you don't eliminate toxins through bowel movements they just recirculate into the bloodstream and make your condition worse. Add more fiber and plenty of water to your diet. This should improve your condition. You may want to consider a mild herbal laxative formula that will not be habit forming. These formulas can be found at most health food stores.

Q. Are there any supplements that I should avoid when trying to prevent future outbreaks?

A. For adult acne, you should not take too much vitamin E or iodine because they can stimulate the sebaceous glands to produce too much oil!

Q. What can I use on open sores on my face that is natural and antibacterial?

A. You can use tea tree oil. The smell is not that pleasant, but it really does a wonderful job because it is a natural antibiotic, antifungal and antiviral agent.

Q. Can you recommend any products on the market that help acne?

A. Yes. Several of my former clients have used Pro-Active. For more information, you can call 1-888-554-3838 (twenty-four hours a day, seven days a week).

Q. Should I avoid the sun?

A. Actually, the sun is wonderful for your skin and a vital source of vitamin D. Just make sure that the sun you get is morning sun, before noon. You only need fifteen to twenty minutes daily.

Q. Will exercise help my skin condition?

A. My recommendation is yes! You need to sweat to release toxins that are stored in your system. I say better out than in when it comes to toxins. The cleaner your body, the clearer your skin becomes.

Q. How big of a part does stress play when it comes to acne?

A. A big part. Stress causes a lot of acidity in the body, which is toxic.

Again, water, exercise, a detox program and dietary changes will help relieve both your stress and your acne. By the way, stress-caused acne is usually found on the chin. In this case, I recommend a good B-complex vitamin that contains pantothenic acid.

Healthy Skin at a Glance

SKIN FOOD

Biotin: 1 mg morning and evening
Manganese: 50 mg evening
Zinc: 30 mg morning and evening
Vitamin C: 1,000 mg morning and evening
Vitamin A: 25,000 IU daily

ADRENAL EXHAUSTION

Do you feel tired, worn out and just plain zapped? It could be that your batteries need recharging. I consider the adrenal glands to be two little batteries that sit on top of your kidneys. They are made up of two parts: the cortex, which is responsible for cortisone production, and the medulla, which secretes adrenaline.

The *cortex* helps to maintain body balance, regulates sugar and carbohydrate metabolism and produces certain sex hormones. The *medulla's* job is to produce epinephrine (otherwise known as adrenaline) and norepinephrine to speed up metabolism in order to cope with stress. When you are under stress, the adrenal glands increase your metabolism to ward off the negative effects.

Adrenal gland function is weakened by consuming too much caffeine and sugar, by vitamin deficiencies and long-term cortico-steroid use and, of course, by too much stress! It is extremely important to keep your batteries charged!

Definition

Adrenal exhaustion is defined as malfunction of the adrenal glands, a pair of glands located on top of the kidneys that release hormones into the bloodstream.

Symptoms

Symptoms include great fatigue, weakness, lethargy, low blood pressure, moodiness, dry skin, poor memory, poor circulation, hypoglycemia or diabetes, poor immune system, cravings for sugar and salt, brittle nails, a feeling of being "driven" and anxiousness.

Causes

The most common causes of adrenal exhaustion are unrelenting stress,

A–type personality and long-term use of cortico-steroid drugs for asthma, arthritis and allergies. As mentioned, too much sugar and caffeine in the diet and a deficiency of vitamins B and C also contribute to the condition. Adrenal exhaustion is common as well during the perimenopausal and menopausal stages of life. It is important to watch for warning signs of this debilitating condition. The main lifestyle change needed for improving the condition is rest, rest and more rest!

WARNING SIGNS OF ADRENAL EXHAUSTION

Severe reactions to odors or certain foods
Recurring yeast infections
Heart palpitations and panic attacks
Dry skin and peeling nails
Clammy hands and soles of feet
Low energy and poor memory
Chronic low back pain
Cravings for salt and sugar

Check your batteries self-test

If you want to see just how well your adrenal glands are performing, try this self-test. First, lie down and rest for five minutes. Then, take your blood pressure. Stand up immediately and take your blood pressure reading once more while standing. If your blood pressure is lower after you stand up, you probably have reduced adrenal gland function, which means your batteries need a charge. The lower the blood pressure reading is from your resting blood pressure, the more severe the low adrenal function. The systolic number (the number on top of the blood pressure reading) normally is about ten points higher when you are standing than when you lie down. A difference of more than ten points should be addressed immediately as it is of extreme importance in the journey back to health. At this point, I recommend that you feed your worn-out adrenals the following supplements to bring them back to full power.

Supplement support for adrenal exhaustion

    ✿   Pantothenic acid is a B vitamin known as an antistress vitamin that plays a role in the production of adrenal hormones. It is very helpful in alleviating anxiety and depression by fortifying the adrenal glands. In addition, pantothenic acid is needed to produce our own natural pain relievers, which include cortisol. This is very important, because pain often goes hand in hand with emotional depletion.

❦ B complex consists of the full spectrum of B vitamins. The B vitamins help to maintain a healthy nervous system.

❦ Vitamin C is required for tissue growth and repair, healthy gums and adrenal gland function. Vitamin C also protects us against infection and strengthens our immunity.

❦ Royal jelly (2 teaspoons daily) is known to be a blessing for the body against asthma, liver disease, skin disorders and immune suppression. This is because it is rich in vitamins, minerals, enzymes and hormones. In addition, it possesses antibiotic and antibacterial properties. It is interesting to note that it naturally contains a high concentration of pantothenic acid.

❦ Astragalus (as directed on the bottle) is an herb that aids adrenal gland function. It also combats fatigue and protects the immune system. This herb played a large part in fortifying and strengthening my body when I battled the Epstein-Barr virus. It truly is a powerful herb in terms of immune boosting.

❦ L-tyrosine is an amino acid that helps to build the body's natural supply of adrenaline and thyroid hormones. It converts to L-dopa, which makes it a safe therapy for depression. If you are on antidepressants or have cancer, you should avoid tyrosine.

❦ Dr. Janet's recommendation: Core Level Adrenal glandular supplement, available from Nutri-West of Florida. Use as directed by your healthcare professional.

CRITICAL SUPPLEMENTS FOR ADRENALS

Vitamin C: 1500 mg of Ester C
Pantothenic acid: 500–2000 mg
B complex: 100 mg
Astragalus
L-tyrosine: 500 mg
Core Level Adrenal glandular supplement
Royal jelly

ADDITIONAL ADRENAL FORTIFIERS

Brewer's yeast
Wheat germ
Flaxseed
Milk thistle
Licorice root
Hawthorne
Gota kola
Siberian ginseng
Daily green drink (Kyo-Green by Wakunaga)
Rest, rest, rest!

Common questions regarding adrenal exhaustion

Q. What dietary considerations will help to strengthen my adrenal glands?

A. Diet is vitally important when it comes to healthy adrenal glands. Make sure that your diet is low in sugar and fats. Also, eat small meals instead of large ones. Stay with fresh foods and cold-water fish like salmon, legumes like lentils, whole grains and brown rice. Cut down on high-sodium foods. Add more potassium-rich foods like potatoes, bananas and avocados. Other helpful foods include almonds, garlic, sunflower seeds, bran and avocado.

Q. Are there any other supplements that can support and strengthen my adrenal glands?

A. I recommend a good digestive enzyme formula that contains the full spectrum of enzymes. This will help to stimulate adrenal cortex production. In addition, I recommend a formula called Core Level Adrenal. (See ordering information found under product sources in back of this book.)

Q. I am under stress that never lets up. How can I protect my adrenal glands from exhaustion?

A. Follow my recommendations and make sure that you add moderated exercise like walking every day. Massage therapy also helps keep adrenals healthy. Massage helps to relieve stored stress and tension in the muscles and helps to clear the adrenal pathways.

Especially for women

If you take care of your adrenal glands, they will take good care of you. This is especially true for women. At the time of perimenopause and beyond, the adrenal glands do double duty by picking up the slack that occurs in ovarian function. The adrenal glands can step in to keep normal balance going if they are strong and not overtaxed by stress, lack of sleep and poor diet. In that case, hormonal free-fall occurs and symptoms are severe. A word to the wise: To be forewarned is to be forearmed. Take care of these glands now, and it will save you much despair later on!

AGING

Even to your old age and gray hairs I am he, I am he who will sustain you. I have made you and I will carry you.

—ISAIAH 46:4, NIV

Poet Robert Browning wrote, "Grow old along with me! The best is yet to be."[1] Why then do we have a culture that tries to stop visible signs of aging at all costs? Maybe because getting older signifies the end of an active life and less vitality mentally, sexually and physically.

In our "youth-worshiping" culture today, so much emphasis is placed on youthful appearance that the plastic surgery business is literally booming, making this once "Hollywood only" group of procedures now available to the average American, complete with convenient finance plans! Unfortunately, our outward appearance does not guarantee happiness in old age.

The truth is, it is the quality of our lives that is important. The inner health of our body, mind and spirit creates either an ageless glow or an old haggard demeanor. The Bible's view on aging is different from Hollywood's. Gray hair and wrinkles are seen as a crown of maturity worthy of honor after enduring life's hardships: "The silver-haired head is a crown of glory, if it is found in the way of righteousness" (Prov. 16:31, NKJV).

Youthfulness is not a chronological age, and age is not the enemy—disease is! The good news is that God made our bodies able to be rejuvenated at any age, thereby giving us more healthy vibrant years. We can slow the aging process by making sure that we maintain the very best internal environment possible to prevent disease.

While it is true that cell age is genetically controlled, disease or illness is most often the result of poor diet, lifestyle and environment, not to mention stress! Research in longevity has shown that there are three main causes of premature aging:

- Enzyme depletion from poor diet and inadequate enzyme supplementation
- Lowered immune response, which sets the stage for disease
- Cell and tissue damage from free radicals

Definition

Aging is the process by which the body matures and grows old or shows signs of growing old that continues throughout the span of life. It is caused by a breakdown in the replacement process of cells that are continually dying.

Antiaging self-quiz

Take this self-quiz to help determine if you are aging faster than necessary.

ANTIAGING SELF-QUIZ

Yes No

☐ ☐   Have you noticed brown spots on the back of your hands or around your eyes and nose?

☐ ☐   Is it more difficult for you to lose weight?

☐ ☐   Do you have frequent indigestion, heartburn or gas after eating a meal?

☐ ☐   Do you have insomnia?

☐ ☐   Do you have heart palpitations or chest pain?

☐ ☐   Do you have poor eyesight?

☐ ☐   Have you experienced hearing loss or ringing in the ears?

☐ ☐   Are you frequently constipated?

☐ ☐   Is your hair turning gray?

❑ ❑   Have you lost height?

❑ ❑   Is your skin becoming dryer or thinner? Are you noticing more moles, bruises or cherry angiomas (red blood blisters)?

❑ ❑   Is your recovery time slow from a cold or flu?

❑ ❑   Do you have poor circulation?

Dietary considerations

Good nutrition is the key to adding years to your life and life to your years. Here are some of the best all-time longevity superfoods as well as those you need to avoid!

First priority is to drink plenty of pure water every day. This will keep you hydrated and help all of your body's systems to work more efficiently. In addition, water will help proper elimination, remove toxins and lessen arthritic pain. It also helps to transport proteins, vitamins, minerals and sugars for assimilation. Water helps the body work at its peak.

Eat fresh seafood at least twice weekly for thyroid health and balance. Nuts, seeds, beans, fiber and essential fatty acids are living nutrients. Enjoy fresh fruits and vegetables—enzyme rich and full of vitamins, minerals and fiber.

Practice caloric reduction. As you age, your body requires fewer calories and also burns calories at a lower rate. In addition, a low-calorie diet has been shown to protect your DNA from damage. This will thereby prevent organ and tissue degeneration. Try to get more "bang for your caloric buck" by eating only high-quality, densely nutritious foods at each meal. For example, lots of fresh fruit and vegetables, organically grown if possible.

Avoid fried foods, red meat, too much caffeine and highly spiced and processed foods.

Supplement support for aging

- Coenzyme Q_{10} for cardiovascular health, periodontal disease or gum problems
- Multivitamin/mineral supplement
- L-glutathione: antioxidant, amino acid that neutralizes radiation and inhibits free radicals
- Gota kola: brain and nervous system health
- Royal jelly: antiaging superfood, great for chronic fatigue and immune health, great source of pantothenic acid
- Lycopene: anticancer antioxidant that reduces the risk of prostate and cervical cancer
- Vitamins C, A and E: antioxidants
- Bilberry: protects against macular degeneration
- Germanium: increases tissue oxygenation, thereby preventing disease

- ❧ Ginkgo biloba: helps restore circulation, improves hearing and vision, improves memory and brain activity
- ❧ Green superfoods: spirulina, chlorella, barley green, kelp and wheatgrass
- ❧ Daily green drink: I recommend Kyo-Green by Wakunaga.
- ❧ Astragalus: for adrenal health, helps to lower blood pressure, improves circulation
- ❧ Reishi, shiitake and maitake mushrooms: power mushrooms that boost immunity, may help prevent cancer and are antiviral and antibacterial
- ❧ Hawthorn berry: protects the heart from free-radical damage, helps the heart pump blood efficiently
- ❧ Plant enzymes: sparks of life; as we age, we become enzyme depleted. Supplementing with plant enzymes improves digestion, thereby enhancing all of our other body functions, i.e. elimination, assimilation, alertness and energy levels.
- ❧ Red ginseng (for men): an adaptogenic herb that provides energy to all body systems, promotes strength, fortifies the body against the effects of stress and fatigue, promotes testosterone production
- ❧ White or American ginseng: helps to stimulate memory centers in the brain
- ❧ Siberian ginseng: supports the glandular system, especially the adrenals, circulation and memory
- ❧ Yogurt or acidophilus: daily for nutrient assimilation, helps to boost friendly bacteria

Emotional health

It is a common fact that people who fill their lives with laughter and share an attitude of optimism live longer and healthier lives. It is important to long life to take time to play and pray!

Common questions about aging

Q. Can exercise really keep me young?

A. Exercise is considered the best "nutrient" of all time. It can prolong fitness at any age. It also helps increase your stamina and circulation, lifts depression and increases joint mobility.

Q. I have arthritis and am afraid to begin an exercise program. I hurt so badly that I don't want to even try it for fear that I will make things worse.

A. I understand. When you are in pain, you don't want to "rock the boat" and make things worse. I recommend that you begin with deep breathing exercises daily (outdoors in the morning is especially good). Deep breathing will help. In addition, stretching exercises will help to limber up the body in the morning. Also, stretching before going to bed at night will help to relax you and promote more restful sleep. You can also begin a walking program. You will be surprised at how great it makes you feel. Begin slowly at first. As you continue, you will see that you can walk faster and for longer periods of time with positive results.

Q. How does my being overweight factor into the aging process? My grandmother lived to be eighty and was overweight. Does it really matter?

A. Let me make this comment. It is widely believed that ten to thirty pounds of extra weight may take two years off your life. Thirty to fifty pounds of extra weight may result in losing four years, and over fifty pounds may take eight years off your life. This is not to mention all of the diseases associated with obesity like diabetes, cancer and arthritis.

Q. I smoke. It is hard for me to quit. Smoking helps to relieve my stress. I want to look younger and feel better. What can I do?

A. Nothing ages you more prematurely than smoking, with the exception of too much sun exposure. Smoking uses up tissue oxygen, which feeds the brain and helps prevent disease. Each cigarette takes eight minutes off your life, one pack a day takes one month off of your life each year, and two packs take ten to fifteen years off your life. In addition, cigarettes contain over four thousand known poisons.[2] I'll discuss natural protocols for helping you quit smoking in the section on smoking.

Q. Can you give me some dietary suggestions that promote longevity?

A. Eat fresh. *If it does not rot or sprout, do without.* Eat as close to the "original garden" as possible. Shop the perimeter of the grocery store where the *live foods* are found.

Health Update — Multivitamins Help!

People over the age of sixty-five who take multivitamins daily suffer only half as many infection-related illnesses as people who do not take vitamins.[3]

❦ Antiaging herb

Boost the antiaging powers of your next meal by adding fresh oregano. Shiow Wang, Ph.D., a scientist at the USDA's Agricultural Research Service, tested the antioxidant action of twenty-seven different culinary herbs and twelve medicinal herbs. All varieties of oregano came out on top. Even more surprising was the fact that oregano's antioxidant activity exceeded that of vitamin E![4]

❦ Vitamin E slows aging.

Researchers believe that vitamin E, taken at the onset of middle age, will slow damage due to aging in the human brain and immune system. Based upon a study in which middle-age mice and old-age mice were fed diets supplemented with vitamin E, the study results showed that normal age-related damage to vital proteins in their brain and immune system cells was delayed and even prevented.[5]

❦ Latest discovery: human growth hormone (HGH)

HGH, also known as somatotropin, is the hormone that regulates growth. When administered to older adults, it reduces fat tissue, rebuilds muscle mass and helps to reverse changes that are associated with aging. Use HGH only under the guidance of your healthcare professional.

Alzheimer's—the Long Good-bye

Older Americans have come to fear that Alzheimer's will cause them to be a caregiver to a loved one or that it will attack them personally. Alzheimer's now has been diagnosed in over four million Americans. This means that 25 to 50 percent of all people over the age of eighty-five are likely to have Alzheimer's disease.[6]

Definition

Alzheimer's is a degenerative disease in which the nerve cells of the brain deteriorate, resulting in impaired memory, thinking and behavior.

Symptoms

The most common symptoms of Alzheimer's disease include disorientation, confusion, memory loss, language impairment, insomnia, irritability, depression and reversion to childhood. The disease is progressive. Death occurs about ten years after diagnosis. Currently there is no known cure, though natural therapies have been successful in slowing brain deterioration.

Causes

Many cases are the result of too many prescription drugs along with nutritional deficiencies. Proper diagnosis is essential. Other factors that contribute to the disease are poor circulation, arteriosclerosis, thyroid malfunction, aluminum toxicity, mercury toxicity, heredity and possible viral connections. Genetic predisposition is present in more than half of the cases.

Dietary considerations

Choosing to eat nutritiously can help to overcome the effects of Alzheimer's disease, especially if you make those choices early in life. The following dietary regimen can be helpful:

Avoid red meats and sugar; eat nuts, eggs and soy. Eat a largely vegetarian diet, choosing organic foods to avoid xenoestrogens from pesticides. Eat foods that block aluminum toxicity such as liver, fish, brown rice, wheat germ and molasses. Drink spring water only as fluoridated water increases aluminum absorption. Eat avocados, poultry and low-fat dairy to boost tryptophan levels. Take vitamins, minerals and nutritional supplements that enhance memory, nourish the brain, protect brain cells and reduce amyloid protein strings to overcome brain damage.

Supplement support for Alzheimer's

     ❦   Vitamin E: 800 IU daily

- ❧ Evening primrose: 500 mg three times daily; feeds the brain
- ❧ Ginkgo biloba: 60 mg three times daily; symptom stabilizer
- ❧ Neuro-Logic by Wakunaga: improves memory and mental acuity
- ❧ Huperzine A: enhances memory retention
- ❧ Daily green drink
- ❧ Phosphatidyl choline: 5,000–10,000 mg; helps overcome brain damage
- ❧ Royal jelly: to improve memory
- ❧ Omega-3 flax oil: nourishes the brain
- ❧ Lysine: 1000 mg to preserve brain cells
- ❧ DHA: natural calcium channel blocker
- ❧ Carnitine: 500 mg two times daily; a brain nutrient, reduces mental decline
- ❧ Coenzyme Q_{10}: 100 mg daily; cellular energy
- ❧ Thiamine (vitamin B_1): 100 mg daily; increases mental power
- ❧ Vitamin B_{12}: 2500 mcg daily; increases mental power
- ❧ Organic wine (in moderation)
- ❧ Purify by Enzymedica: take as directed to help overcome brain damage by reducing amyloid strings

ALZHEIMER'S AND VITAMIN E

In a study that included patients with moderately severe Alzheimer's, Alzheimer's progression was slowed by high doses of vitamin E—as much as 2,000 IU of vitamin E daily. As a result, these patients had a six- to seven-month delay in the progression of the dementia caused by the disease.

The normal daily dose of vitamin E is 30 IU. Higher doses should be taken under the supervision of a healthcare professional.[7]

Lifestyle choices

Since higher than normal mercury levels have been found in the brains of people with Alzheimer's disease, mercury exposure, which occurs mainly through dental amalgams, should not be overlooked as a potential contributor to Alzheimer's disease. Mercury toxicity releases into the brain and affects brain health. Consider removing silver amalgam dental fillings.

Most biological dentists have amalgam removal protocols that are followed before, during and after the removal process that involve chelators and cleansers. These protocols are necessary to keep your system from reacting adversely to the removal of this heavy metal. See page 146 for a protocol to follow when going through amalgam removal.

Again, drink only spring water. Fluoridated water increases absorption of aluminum into the body from deodorants, pots and pans, dandruff shampoo, antacids, salt, buffered aspirin and fast food. Be an informed consumer.

Health Update — Help in Preventing Alzheimer's

ESTROGEN: MEMORY PILL?

Studies suggest that postmenopausal women who take estrogen replacement therapy (ERT) develop Alzheimer's disease at a lower rate than women who do not. This is because estrogen may help the brain withstand Alzheimer's by promoting the growth and branching of nerve cells in the brain and by improving blood flow and circulation there.[8]

CAUTION: It is important to note that estrogen increases the risk for breast, uterine and ovarian cancer over time. Women with a family history of any of these hormone-related cancers should not take estrogen. If you do take estrogen, take natural estrogen, and only after having your hormone levels assayed by saliva or serum (blood work) to verify that a deficiency is present.

NSAIDS CAN HELP

A study has found that the use of NSAIDS (nonsteroidal anti-inflammatory drugs) such as ibuprofen and naproxen reduced the risk of Alzheimer's disease 30 to 60 percent. This leads researchers to believe that inflammation in the brain may play a part in the disease. Aspirin and acetaminophen were found not to have any positive impact in the study.[9]

ANDROPAUSE (MALE MENOPAUSE)

Even though men's hormonal fluctuations are not as pronounced as women's during midlife, the male body needs extra attention during this time of life. Formally known as the "male midlife crisis," andropause clearly is a time where many men feel that they have lost their vitality, strength and youth as their muscle mass, energy and sexual performance decline. If you are in andropause, natural remedies can be an effective way to reenergize every area of your life. Prostate health must be addressed. Diet must be improved and lifestyle changes must be made in order to prevent degenerative disease.

You can restore your energy, stamina and sexual satisfaction. Consider andropause as a time to "pause" and reevaluate your diet and lifestyle. Get a complete medical checkup with all of the appropriate health screenings. And use the following recommendations to keep you healthy as you embark on the second half of your journey of life.

Definition

Andropause occurs around the age of forty when testosterone levels begin to decline. These levels continue to fall about 10 percent each decade thereafter.[10]

Symptoms

Symptoms of andropause include fatigue, head hair growth slowed, ear hair increased, loss of muscle mass, frequent urination, postural changes, weight gain around the middle, low sex drive and depression.

Dietary considerations
Limit red meats, fried foods, full-fat dairy foods, caffeine and sugar. Brewer's yeast, seeds, nuts and oysters are good food sources for sexual health.

Supplement support for andropause
- Tribulus terrestris
- For impotence: ginkgo biloba liquid extract three times daily
- For prostate health: saw palmetto, pygeum zinc. Limit or eliminate alcohol (beer especially elevates DHT levels).
- To increase muscle mass: whey protein shake in the morning; L-glutamine stimulates your own growth hormones.
- A daily "green drink," like Kyo-Green

Lifestyle choices
Exercise is a vital part of male sexuality, improving frequency, satisfaction and performance.

Stress management is vital for sexual health. Stress zaps your adrenal glands. Healthy adrenals are needed at andropause to prevent fatigue and burnout. Adrenal exhaustion in men is linked to depression and anxiety attacks. Limit coffee, and make an effort to get enough hours of sleep each night. Watch your sugar intake. Adrenal support recommendations include B complex, adrenal glandular formula, royal jelly and pantothenic acid.

Tips for extending men's healthy lives
Men can add years to their lives by knowing how to age properly. Here are six tips by experts for extending men's healthy lives:[11]

1. Have a personal physician, someone you've seen when your temperature is below 102 and you don't need crutches. "Then you've formed a relationship, so if something does happen, there's somebody who knows you."

2. Make close friends. Social interaction and strong friendships keep coming up in research as important predictors of longer and happy lives.

3. Learn how to express anger constructively as opposed to destructively.

4. Know the signs of heart attack and stroke. Men can't change their generally higher death rates from cardiovascular disease, but they can boost their individual survival odds as well as reduce their risk through diet, exercise and periodic blood tests.

5. Let go of the notion that you're invincible or omnipotent. Reducing stress is not a sign of weakness!

6. Be careful. No, you don't have to buy a hardhat for hanging pictures in the hallway, but you shouldn't be climbing a shaky ladder either. A cast doesn't make anyone look tough, and the causes of death where men outpace women the most are injuries, suicide and liver disease, often the result of excessive drinking. So wear a seatbelt, don't drive drunk and do some stretching before that workout.

Health Update   Tomatoes Help Prevent Prostate Cancer

A study of almost fifty thousand men found that those who ate two or more servings of cooked tomato products a week had one-third less risk of developing prostate cancer than those who rarely ate cooked tomato products. Tomatoes contain a high amount of lycopene, an antioxidant. Other sources of lycopene include cabbage, broccoli, carrots and soybeans.[12]

ANGINA

Because angina symptoms can closely parallel symptoms of a heart attack, let me begin by warning you *always* to seek medical attention when experiencing symptoms of a heart attack. CALL 911 IMMEDIATELY. Those symptoms are deep, severe pain in the chest that radiates to the left arm, neck, jaw or between the shoulder blades, shortness of breath, nausea and vomiting.

Definition
Angina is pain or pressure in the chest that lasts for several minutes and can radiate into the neck or arm.

Symptoms
Symptoms include sudden, intense chest pains, vise-grip-like in nature and lasting thirty to sixty seconds. Angina can be a warning sign of an impending heart attack or other cardiac event. It can be brought on by partially closed arteries, causing the heart to work harder and painfully. Overexertion, cold weather and, of course, stress can also trigger angina.

Dietary considerations
Follow a vegetarian diet. Drinking a glass of red wine after dinner can reduce stress and increase HDL. You should also drink green tea and plenty of nonchlorinated water. When cooking, use onions and garlic; you can also take Kyolic Garlic daily.

Supplement support for angina

- Coenzyme Q_{10}: 100 mg daily
- Magnesium: 400–800 mg daily
- Omega-3 or flax oil

- Gingko biloba
- Carnitine

Lifestyle choices

- Exercise daily (walking is very good).
- Do deep-breathing exercises.
- Stop smoking (please see smoking section).

Emergency measures to help stop a heart attack:

- Cayenne liquid under the tongue: 30 drops
- One teaspoon cayenne powder under the tongue
- Chew one aspirin for symptoms of a heart attack to help prevent death and reduce arterial blockage

ANXIETY

Nearly 1.6 percent of American adults suffer symptoms that range from mild anxiety to full-blown panic attacks caused by a form of anxiety.[13] Anxiety-related symptoms send millions of Americans to doctors' offices or emergency rooms each year.[14] Anxiety tends to develop as a result of emotional or physical stress, whether it be from a childhood trauma, divorce, financial problems, unrelenting relationship problems or job pressure. Some anxiety conditions seem to be hereditary in nature, running in families. Anxiety disorder affects twice as many women as men.[15]

Definition

Anxiety, which is a combination of physical and emotional conditions that mirror the flight-or-fight response, can be *acute,* producing panic attacks, or *chronic,* producing symptoms that make life difficult. Anxiety conditions not properly treated can pave the way for high blood pressure, heart attacks, low immunity and cancer.

Symptoms

Symptoms include fear, irritability, insomnia, high blood pressure, head and neck aches, stiff and tight muscles, dizziness, loss of appetite, stomach problems, constipation, ulcer, colitis, rapid heartbeat and shallow breathing.

Dietary considerations

Avoid sugar, caffeine and alcohol. These tax your adrenal glands. Feed your adrenal glands with beans, nuts, whole grains and royal jelly. To protect your nerves, add to your diet foods rich in magnesium like kelp, soy foods, wheat germ, bran and nuts. Add foods rich in vitamin C, such as cherries, broccoli, peppers and green leafy vegetables. Add foods rich in calcium, such as almonds, sesame seeds, soy foods and low-fat dairy products.

Supplement support for anxiety

Vitamin, herb and mineral therapy will calm, rebuild and rebalance body chemistry and boost adrenal glands. The following supplements can help:

- GABA: daily and during an attack, 750 mg as needed; acts as a natural tranquilizer (always take with vitamin B_6)
- 5-HTP: 50 mg
- Magnesium: 400 mg at bedtime
- Passionflower extract
- Adrenal glandular supplement
- B complex
- Ashwagandha
- Valerian extract
- L-theanine (derived from green tea)—may be taken with GABA
- AC-24 (twenty-four-hour anxiety control formula available from the Pain and Stress Center)
- Dr. Janet's Balanced by Nature Tranquility

Lifestyle choices

- Massage
- Deep-breathing exercises
- Walking or other forms of exercise
- Prayer

Bible wisdom

The Bible teaches us to bring our anxieties to God: "Casting all your care upon Him, for He cares for you" (1 Pet. 5:7, NKJV). We can learn to rest in the loving care of God as we meditate on His promises and cultivate relationship with Him.

And Jesus declared:

> Do not be anxious for your life, as to what you shall eat, or what you shall drink; nor for your body as to what you shall put on. Is not life more than food, and the body than clothing? Look at the birds of the air; that they do not sow, neither do they reap, nor gather into barns, and yet your heavenly Father feeds them. Are you not worth much more than they? And which of you by being anxious can add a single cubit to his life's span?...Do not be anxious then, saying, "What shall we eat?" or "What shall we drink?" or "With what shall we clothe ourselves?" For all these things the Gentiles eagerly seek; for your heavenly Father knows that you need all these things. But seek first His kingdom and His righteousness; and all these things shall be added to you. Therefore do not be anxious for tomorrow; for tomorrow will care for itself. Each day has enough trouble of its own.
>
> —MATTHEW 6:25–27, 31–34, NAS

ARTERIOSCLEROSIS

Natural medicine believes that this condition is not only preventable, but it is also reversible. A B$_6$ deficiency and a high-fat diet are thought to be the major causes instead of high cholesterol as previously thought. As with many health conditions, stress plays a part in the development of arteriosclerosis.

Other factors that contribute to the disease are obesity, smoking, diabetes, alcohol consumption and excess sodium and caffeine in the diet, along with poor diet and a sedentary lifestyle. When arteriosclerosis occurs, the flow of blood is blocked or hindered from reaching the heart, which can damage the circulatory system.

Definition
Arteriosclerosis can be defined as the thickening and decreased elasticity of the arterial walls.

Symptoms
Symptoms include leg cramps, high blood pressure, cold hands and feet, blurred vision, mental decline and respiratory problems.

Dietary considerations
Add fiber to your diet. Eat plenty of fruits and vegetables for their antioxidant benefit; they help to keep arteries clear and free of clogs. Vegetarians have less heart disease. Have a glass of red wine at dinner or shortly after. Avoid red meat, dairy products, sugar and fried foods. Reduce coffee intake; consider replacing it with roasted dandelion tea, which has the taste of coffee and is wonderful for your liver.

Supplement support for arteriosclerosis
- Garlic capsules: four times daily (Kyolic)
- Vitamin B complex
- Red wine (one glass daily)
- Flax oil
- Coenzyme Q$_{10}$
- Ester C: 500 mg three times daily
- Magnesium chloride: 400–800 mg daily
- Vitamin E: 400 IU
- Chromium: 200 mcg daily
- Ginkgo biloba
- Milk thistle extract
- Carnitine

Lifestyle choices
There are several lifestyle choices that you can make to help prevent or battle arteriosclerosis. Taking a walk after dinner or walking on the treadmill for aerobic exercise will help increase circulation. So will stopping smoking. If you are obese or overweight, begin a weight-reducing plan that you can live with.

| *Health Update* | Cutting the Risk of Heart Disease |

ELEVATED HOMOCYSTEINE: RISK FACTOR
FOR CARDIOVASCULAR DISEASE

Medical journals now recognize that elevated level of homocysteine is a risk factor for cardiovascular disease. Homocysteine can cause abnormal blood clot formation inside the arteries, which leads to stroke and heart attacks. In addition, elevated homocysteine levels cause atherosclerosis. A simple blood test will reveal elevated levels.

The following supplements can lower homocysteine levels safely and effectively:

- Folic acid: 800 mcg
- Vitamin B_{12}: 300 mcg
- Trimethylglycine: 500 mg

ARTHRITIS

Contrary to popular belief, arthritis is not a single disease with a single cause. The causes vary and can be attributed to emotional problems, viral or bacterial infections or a history of sports-related injuries. The most common form of arthritis is osteoarthritis, which affects more then twenty-one million Americans.[16] That number is expected to grow as more and more of us are living longer lives.

Rheumatoid arthritis (RA) is found in about seven million Americans, with most sufferers being female.[17] This is a more serious condition because it is a chronic inflammatory disease with far-reaching damage that includes bone, cartilage and inflammation of the heart, lungs and blood vessels. Stress and adrenal exhaustion play a big part in the onset of RA. Food allergies and liver malfunction have also been implicated.

Americans ingest millions of NSAID medications like Motrin (ibuprofen) to stop the pain. But NSAIDS have risks and side effects, which include gastrointestinal bleeding along with the further progression of the disease.

Arthritis cripples many of us as we age, but it does not have to. There are natural ways to keep your joints pain free and supple.

Definition

Arthritis is inflammation of a joint with pain and stiffness.

Symptoms

The most common symptoms of arthritis are pain, swelling, stiffness and diminished range of motion. It often appears in the weight-bearing joints: the hips, knees and spine. The first sign of the disease is usually morning stiffness and pain that worsens with movement and activity.

Dietary considerations

Eat a low-fat diet with plenty of fresh fruits and vegetables, olive oil, cold-water fish, cherries, garlic, onions and green tea. Individuals with arthritis should avoid fried foods, dairy, alcohol, sugar and caffeine. They should also avoid allergy foods: corn, wheat, rye, eggs and nightshades (eggplant, chocolate, tomatoes, potatoes, sodas and peppers).

Supplement support for arthritis

The following supplements can aid overall health and specifically allow the body to reduce the inflammation and pain caused by arthritis:

- Dr. Janet's Balanced by Nature Glucosamine Cream
- Glucosamine sulfate: 1500 mg
- Enzymedica's Purify
- DLPA: 1000 mg (for pain)
- Bromelain: 1500 mg daily
- Ester C: 3000 mg daily (for collagen production)
- Pantothenic acid
- Royal jelly (for adrenal rejuvenation)
- MSM: 1000 mg daily
- Chondroitin
- Alfalfa tablets
- Daily green drink (Kyo-Green)
- Turmeric

Lifestyle choices

- Dry sauna
- Massage therapy
- Deep breathing
- Stretching exercises
- Therapeutic baths

Health Update — Wobenzym for Arthritis

Over 100 million people use Wobenzym daily! This best-selling, over-the-counter product is second only to aspirin in Germany. Over fifty clinical studies confirm Wobenzym's positive findings in cases of osteoarthritis, rheumatoid arthritis, reduction in C-reactive protein, and sprains and strains.[18] Healing properties include:

- Helps to control joint inflammation
- Supports healthy blood flow
- Mobilizes the immune system
- Speeds recovery from sprains and strains

Joint Health Quiz

Your answers to the following questions will help assess your risk for arthritis.

Step 1: What's Your Risk?

Yes No

❑   ❑   Are you forty-five years of age or older?

❑   ❑   Have you ever had an injury to your knee(s) severe enough to put you in bed, to force you to use a cane, crutch or brace or to require surgery?

❑   ❑   Are you more than 10 pounds overweight?

❑   ❑   Do you currently participate in (or have you in the past) more than three hours a day of strenuous physical activities such as bending, lifting and carrying items on a regular basis?

❑   ❑   Did you have hip problems that caused you to limp as a child?

Step 2: What Are Your Symptoms?

Yes No

❑   ❑   Has a doctor ever told you that you have arthritis?

❑   ❑   During the past twelve months, have you had pain, aching, stiffness or swelling in or around a joint?

❑   ❑   In a typical month, were these symptoms present daily for at least half of the days?

❑   ❑   Do you have pain in your knee(s) or hip(s) when climbing stairs or walking two or three blocks (one-quarter mile) on level ground?

❑   ❑   Do you have daily pain or stiffness in your hand joints?

❑   ❑   Are you presently limited in any way in activities because of joint symptoms (pain, aching, stiffness and loss of motion)?

Step 3: Because of Joint Symptoms, Use the Listed Ratings to Assess Your Ability to Do the Following:

(0 = no difficulty, 1 = some difficulty, 2 = much difficulty, 3 = unable to do)

____ Dress yourself, including shoelaces and buttons

____ Stand up from a straight, armless chair

____ Get in and out of a car

____ Open a car door

Health Update   **Glucosamine Relieves Arthritis Symptoms**

In a recent study, glucosamine sulfate was effective in relieving joint pain associated with osteoarthritis. Glucosamine's pain-relieving effects may be due to its cartilage-rebuilding properties. These benefits are not seen with simple analgesics and are of particular benefit. The study concluded that glucosamine can be used as an alternative to anti-inflammatory drugs and analgesics.[19]

Choose the appropriate dose of glucosamine for your use from the following information.

Body weight:

- 120 pounds or less: 1,000 mg glucosamine; 800 mg chondroitin
- 120–200 pounds: 1,500 mg glucosamine; 1,200 mg chondroitin
- 200 pounds and over: 2,000 mg glucosamine; 1,600 mg chondroitin

How to take: Divide doses in half, and take one-half in the morning and one-half in the evening with food.

ASTHMA

This illness literally "takes your breath away." Asthma is a severe respiratory allergy reaction. It is the most serious chronic illness among children under the age of ten. It is estimated that 3 to 5 percent of our population is affected by this disorder. There has been a 50 percent increase in diagnosed cases in the last several years, with a suspected link to the increase of environmental pollutants.[20]

Studies show that there are common triggers that precipitate an attack of asthma in children. The most common trigger is stress. Other triggers include smoke, food dyes, certain food allergies, molds, pet dander, chemical toxins and respiratory infections. In adults, asthma triggers or precipitators are adrenal gland exhaustion, constipation, low thyroid function and hypoglycemia.

Definition

Asthma is a respiratory disorder causing attacks of wheezing and breathlessness.

Symptoms

Symptoms include difficulty breathing, feeling as if you are "starved for air," wheezing, coughing, choking, heart palpitations and panic.

ASTHMA SELF-TEST

Yes No

☐   ☐   Are you often anxious? (Fear of suffocation gives many asthmatics chronic anxiety.)

☐   ☐   Do you have a rapid pulse? (You may be responding to a lack of oxygen or may have an underlying allergy.)

☐   ☐   Do you need more than one breath to finish each sentence when speaking? (Many asthmatics need to breathe in mid-sentence.)

☐   ☐   Do you make a wheezing sound when you breathe? (Wheezing is a sign of inflammation, narrowing of the airway or excess production of mucus.)

☐   ☐   Are you breathing wrong? (Asthmatics tend to breathe from the chest, lifting their shoulders as they inhale instead using the diaphragm to lift the belly.)

☐   ☐   Are you in pain? (Because they use the wrong muscles to breathe, asthmatics often have back, chest or abdominal pain.)[21]

Dietary considerations

Begin a largely vegetarian diet. Green leafy vegetables are especially good because of their high magnesium content, which helps to relax bronchial muscles. Drink plenty of water with lemon to thin mucous secretions. Have your food sensitivities identified. Consider allergy testing. This will help you avoid your personal asthma triggers, thereby reducing the frequency of your attacks. Reduce sodium and starchy foods in your diet. Asthmatics have more frequent attacks when they consume high amounts of sodium (salty) foods. To cut down on mucus production, avoid dairy products. Avoid soft drinks, caffeine, fried foods, sulfites, MSG and sugary foods.

Supplement support for asthma

- ❧ Vitamin C: 3000 mg
- ❧ Quercetin: 1000–2000 mg daily

- Vitamin E: 400 IU with 200 mcg selenium
- Coenzyme Q$_{10}$: 100 mg
- Magnesium: 400 mg
- Bromelain: 500 mg
- Daily green drink
- Lobelia extract, placed under the tongue to relax the chest constriction
- Reishi mushroom extract
- Echinacea and goldenseal: to thin mucus
- Astragalus: to strengthen the immune system
- Gingko biloba: to help ease breathing
- Royal jelly: for adrenal gland help

Lifestyle choices

- Apply a hot ginger compress to the chest.
- Massage therapy eases stress and relaxes muscle tension.
- Deep-breathing exercises create proper breathing technique.
- Walk every day, or ride your bicycle.
- Avoid tobacco smoke. If you smoke, STOP!
- Vacuum your home often.
- Use laundry detergent free of perfumes and dyes.

Dr. Janet's Special Recommendations

- B.E.#3 Breath-Ease by Ancient Formulas (1-800-543-3026)
- Clear Lungs by Ridge Crest Herbals (www.ridgecrestherbals.com)

ATHLETE'S FOOT AND OTHER SKIN INFECTIONS

This condition can be persistent and annoying. It is characterized by moist, weepy, red patches on the body (feet and groin are most common areas). A major cause of fungal infections is long courses of antibiotic therapy that kill friendly digestive flora, which in turn lowers immunity and allows fungal infections to take hold. Strengthening the immune system will help to curb future occurrences.

Definition

Athlete's foot is a fungal infection in which the skin between the toes cracks, blisters and peels.

Symptoms

Symptoms include moist, weepy or dry scaly patches that are cracked, tender or bleeding.

Causes

Athlete's foot or toenail fungus can be caused by poorly fitting shoes that are nonporous, not allowing perspiration to evaporate. This results in candida albicans/yeast overgrowth.

Dietary considerations for athlete's foot

Follow the eating plan as outlined on the section on candidiasis. Avoid sugar, soft drinks, red meats, dairy and wheat. Reduce all carbohydrates. Eat plenty of cultured foods to promote healthy bowel flora. Keep the diet simple with plenty of fresh vegetables and fruits. Eat enough protein each day from poultry, whey protein, eggs, soy foods and seafood to boost immunity.

Supplement support for fungal infections

- Olive leaf extract capsules
- Oregano oil capsules
- Garlic capsules: three capsules daily
- Evening primrose capsules
- Acidophilus: take before meals
- Protease (a digestive enzyme)
- Zinc: 30 mg daily
- Lysine: 1000 mg daily

Lifestyle choices

Try one or both of the following foot soaks:

- Athlete's foot soak: A sea salt soak—if possible, go to the beach and soak in the ocean.

- Use a basin with tea tree oil, twenty-five drops in warm water. Soak for twenty minutes. Towel dry, apply baking soda and put clean socks on before bed each night. In the morning, dab tea tree oil between the toes with a cotton ball; soak feet in apple cider vinegar and water on alternate days.

Health Update — Common Causes of Athlete's Foot

Most cases of athlete's foot are caused by candida, the same yeast that causes vaginal infections and/or by T. rubrum, another type of fungus. Following the dietary considerations for candidiasis can be helpful to relieve this condition.

BLADDER INFECTION

This painful condition affects many women in America. Over 75 percent of American women have at least one urinary tract infection in a ten-year period.[22] Many women suffer at least once a year from the infection. There are several causes, which include staph, strep, *E. coli* bacterium, overuse of antibiotics, menopausal tissue changes, lack of fluids, poor elimination and stress. But most often, the *E. coli* bacterium that travels up the urethra is the culprit. If the infection is not addressed, the kidneys can be infected as well, making it a much more serious condition that can even lead to kidney failure. It is essential to begin attacking the infection at the first sign of infection.

Definition
Bladder infection is an inflammation of the bladder usually associated with *E. coli* bacterium.

Symptoms
Symptoms include painful, frequent and urgent urination with pain in the lower back and abdominal area, chills and fever as the body tries to fight the infection. The urine is usually cloudy with a strong smell and, occasionally, with traces of blood. Symptoms are very uncomfortable and life disrupting.

Dietary considerations
During the acute stage, take 2 tablespoons of apple cider vinegar and honey in water in the morning.

To alkalize your system, changing your body's pH, eat watermelon and drink Kyo-Green (a green drink), celery juice and cucumber juice. Avoid chocolate, spinach, sugar, dairy and red meat, which acidify the system. Drink eight to ten glasses of purified water and diluted fruit juice (especially unsweetened cranberry) daily to flush your system. Eat a yeast-free diet. (See the section on candida.)

Supplement support for bladder infection
- Uva ursi capsules
- Vitamin C
- Acidophilus liquid
- Goldenseal-echinacea extract
- Cranberry capsules
- Grapefruit extract capsules

Lifestyle choices
- Limit the use of a diaphragm.
- Urinate as soon as possible after intercourse.
- Drink a glass of water with 1 teaspoon of baking soda added.
- Place a warm castor oil pack on the abdomen.
- Place a ginger pack on the kidneys.

BRAIN DRAIN

The key to avoiding dullness of mind, or worse, is to replenish and rejuvenate the brain. If you experience memory lapses, moodiness, depression, spaciness, poor concentration, anxiety and forgetfulness, you are not alone. In today's world, stress is taking a toll on our brain health and balance. We are overworked, burned out, stressed out and lacking desperately in "down time."

Stress depletes the brain and body of amino acids, the building blocks of protein, and of potassium. A deficiency of amino acids and potassium contributes to mental burnout. You must feed your brain to replenish and restore optimal brain function. Brain nutrients can quickly improve brain performance, correcting many emotional and physical symptoms as well.

Definition

Located in the skull, the brain is the body's command center. Everyday tasks can overwhelm the brain if it does not receive the proper nutrients for optimal health, causing many of the symptoms mentioned above.

Dietary considerations

The brain thrives on the same healthy foods as the rest of the body, including eggs, olive oil, fruits (especially apples), leafy green vegetables and whole grains like brown rice. For brain health, it is good to avoid sugar, alcohol and tobacco.

Supplement support for the brain

- Omega-3 oils
- DHA oils
- EPA oils
- Wheat germ
- Brewer's yeast
- Lecithin
- Royal jelly
- Gingko biloba
- GABA (take with vitamin B_6)
- 5-HTP at bedtime to boost serotonin level
- Glutamine
- Glycine
- Magnesium gel caps, 800 mg, or 10–15 drops liquid magnesium chloride
- Flax oil
- Coenzyme Q_{10} with vitamin E: 60–100 mg daily
- B complex

Lifestyle choices

- Exercise consistently.
- Learn to do deep-breathing exercises.
- Listen to soothing music.
- Work crossword puzzles or other "mental games" to build more brain circuits.

Amino acids for brain and body function

Amino acids are vital to proper brain function. Understanding your brain function will give you a more comprehensive picture of how various amino acids are effective for the treatment of pain, stress, anxiety and depression. Your body needs and uses basic nutrients every day. These include vitamins, minerals, proteins, carbohydrates and fats. If you were to take the water and fat out of your body, 75 percent of what remains is protein. Muscles, cell membranes, enzymes and neurotransmitters in the brain are all proteins.

Amino acids are involved in basic cellular energy production. They are the building blocks of proteins and are found in every tissue of the body. As a result, amino acids have more diverse functions than other nutrients. They contribute to the formation of muscles, neurotransmitters, enzymes, antibodies and receptors. Therefore, amino acid imbalances can manifest as a variety of symptoms and metabolic disorders.

SYMPTOMS OF AMINO ACID DEFICIENCIES

Behavioral disorders	Rheumatoid arthritis	Osteoarthritis
Candida infections	Digestive disorders	Muscle weakness
Aggression	Chronic pain	Poor concentration
Immune system disorders	Chronic allergies	Food, chemical sensitivity
Vitamin and mineral deficiencies	Mental confusion	Neurological disorders
Eating disorders	Digestive disorder	Anxiety
Hypoglycemia	Learning disorders	ADD/hyperactivity
Diabetes	Depression	Cancer
Chronic fatigue (emotional and physical)	Mood swings	Fear
	Panic attacks	Headaches
Phobias	Cardiovascular disease	Irritable bowel syndrome
	Seizures	Substance abuse

Determine specific amino acid deficiencies by having a twenty-panel amino acid blood test (fasting plasma) drawn. Consult an orthomolecular healthcare professional or call the Pain and Stress Center (800-669-2256).[23]

Health Update   **Brain Drain**
Proverb

"A strain on the brain is felt mostly as a drain."[24]

Balancing the brain

While writing this book, I came across an interesting article entitled "The Brain's Balancing Act" that was very informative.[25] In essence, the article said that working either the left or right side of your brain too hard can wreak havoc with your whole body. By stimulating the underused portion of your brain, balance can be restored. When your brain is in balance, your well-being increases, and your health receives immediate benefit. Let's examine this theory.

The left side of our brain sees individual parts that make up a whole. It organizes, analyzes and rationalizes information. It is also the verbal side of your brain, responding to speech and using words to name and describe things. It keeps track of time and thinks in terms of consequences.

The right brain addresses emotions and is affected by music, touch and body language. It follows hunches and feelings rather than logic. It is the visual side of your brain responding to pictures, colors and shapes. Overreliance on one side can create frustration and eventual brain burnout.

What affects the brain also affects the body. The results of brain burnout can lead to physical problems such as insomnia, headaches and fatigue. The reason for this is that a body cannot be healthy if the brain is not in balance. The following chart developed by Ann McCombs, D.O., who works with hemispericity, shows her findings that certain symptoms indicate a brain imbalance. Most symptoms are left- or right-side specific. There are, however, some symptoms that could indicate a strain of either side

SYMPTOMS OF BRAIN IMBALANCE

Overtaxed Right Brain
Staring off into space
Feelings of panic
Difficulty paying attention
Feeling overly sensitive and emotional

For Right Brain Relief
Work on a crossword puzzle.
Organize your closet.
Play a game of logic (chess).
Learn new software.
Develop a personal budget.

Overtaxed Left Brain
Feelings of worry
Difficulty communicating
Inability to follow a schedule
Difficult problem solving

For Left Brain Relief
Dance.
Listen to music.
Cook or make a gourmet dish.
Play with your children.
Take a walk outdoors.

BREAST DISEASE

Once a woman finds a suspicious breast lump, her natural reaction is fear. But here are the facts: The majority of breast lumps are not cancerous. Although all breast lumps need medical evaluation, you should take comfort in the fact that chances are that any breast lump you may discover is one of several types of harmless lumps that occur in breast tissue. As a rule, benign lumps are usually tender and are moveable while cancerous lumps are usually painless and fixed or do not move freely.[26]

Definition

Breast disease can be defined as a tumor, cyst or infection found in the breast tissue.

Symptoms

The most common cause of breast lumps is fibrocystic breast disease. It is characterized by cysts and thickening of the milk glands. Symptoms include lumpiness in the breast and tenderness that becomes more pronounced just before the menstrual cycle. This condition typically affects women between the ages of thirty and fifty because this is when there is a higher incidence of hormonal fluctuations and imbalances. The primary imbalance is estrogen dominance, which seems to "feed" cysts or multiply their occurrence.

Medical diagnosis

There are four basic types of breast lumps:

- Lipoma—a benign, painless tumor made up of fatty tissue. Usually considered harmless, it has the potential to become malignant.
- Fibroadenoma—commonly found in women twenty years of age and older. It is usually a rubbery, firm and painless mass commonly found on the upper portion of the breast.
- Cystosarcoma—a fast-growing benign tumor that grows in the connective tissue of the breast. In rare instances, it can become malignant.
- Carcinoma of the breast—can include a dark discharge from the nipple, a dimpled area of skin that can be seen directly over the lump. Malignant breast lumps are usually the size of a pea and are hard to the touch. In most cases only one breast is affected at a time.

DIAGNOSTIC METHODS FOR BREAST DISEASE

Mammography	Thermography
Needle aspiration	Surgical biopsy
Ultrasound	

Dietary considerations

Eat a low-fat, high-fiber diet, whole grains, garlic, onions, fresh fruits, yogurt and legumes. Cruciferous vegetables such as broccoli, cabbage and Brussels sprouts contain indoles, which help to protect breast tissue from estrogen metabolites (by-products of estrogen that can contribute to estrogen dominance). Focus on soy foods, which help to bind up bad estrogen. Avoid animal and dairy products, and limit sugar, fried foods, white flour and refined foods. Also limit coffee, tea and other sources of caffeine, which is directly linked to fibrocystic disease. Limit alcohol consumption as well.

Supplement support for breast disease

- Isoflavones: soy-based foods or capsules that help protect breasts from tumor formation
- Natural Progesterone Cream: Dr. Janet's Woman's Balance Formula to correct estrogen dominance
- Evening primrose oil: essential fatty acid shown to reduce breast lumps because of its anti-prostaglandin agents.[27]

❦   Vitamin E: 800–1,200 IU daily, an antioxidant and hormone modulator. Studies have found that vitamin E dramatically improves breast tenderness.

❦   Vitamin A: 10,000–15,000 IU daily, reduces breast pain and is a free radical scavenger; helps breast ducts function optimally[28]

❦   Kelp: 1,000–2,000 IU daily, a rich source of iodine. Breast disease has been associated with iodine deficiency.

❦   Indoles: phytochemicals that negate the effect of bad circulating estrogen to prevent further growth of breast tumors

Health Update   Natural Breast Cancer Prevention

Indole-3 Carbinol (I3C), derived from cruciferous vegetables, inhibits estrogen metabolites that are associated with breast and endometrial cancer. It is a powerful antioxidant that protects DNA and makes cells resistant to damage. Studies have shown this vegetable extract to stop human cancer cells from growing by 54 to 61 percent and that it provokes the diseased cells to self-destruct, a process known as apoptosis.

I3C protects against the environmental carcinogen dioxin. It works in estrogen-receptor, negative-breast-cancer cells. In addition, it increases the conversion of estradiol to the weaker estrogen with a 50 percent reduction noted within one week. Under laboratory conditions, it inhibited the growth of MCF7 breast cancer cells better than tamoxifen. The dose is 200 mg twice daily. It is activated by stomach acid, so it is not to be taken with antacids.

Lifestyle choices

❦   Hot moist packs on breast
❦   Warm castor oil packs
❦   Regular massage to manage stress

BRONCHITIS

This condition can be acute or chronic, leaving you more susceptible to respiratory infections. It can be similar to a chest cold, or it can be stubborn and difficult to treat, lasting for weeks or months. It can be brought on by stress, which lowers the immune system, or develop from exposure to cigarette smoke or chemicals.

Definition

Bronchitis can be defined as an inflammation of the airways (bronchi) of the lungs.

Symptoms

Bronchitis sometimes starts as a cold virus, but subsequently moves deep inside the chest with symptoms that include headache, fever, body aches, lethargy, hacking cough and mucous-clogged airways, which can cause breathing difficulty, nausea and weight loss due to decreased appetite.

Supplement support for bronchitis

- ❦ Echinacea
- ❦ Cordyceps
- ❦ Vitamins A, C and E with selenium
- ❦ NAC (N-acetyl cysteine) to thin mucus
- ❦ Beta glucan
- ❦ Grapefruit seed extract capsules
- ❦ Rub white flower oil on chest
- ❦ Oil of oregano

Dietary considerations

Reishi mushrooms are helpful for bronchitis. Fresh lemon and water are also helpful, and you can make a vegetable broth to drink throughout the day. Your daily green drink will help as well.

You can make your own cough syrup from six onions, ½ cup honey and a pinch of cayenne pepper. Cook in a saucepan on low heat for about two hours. Strain the mixture, removing the onions. Take 1 tablespoon every two to three hours as needed.

Lifestyle choices

- ❦ Ginger and cayenne compresses may be applied to the chest to help loosen mucus.
- ❦ Practice deep-breathing exercises.
- ❦ Get a little morning sun and fresh air each day.
- ❦ Have a brisk massage.

BURNS

Burns can range from the sting of summer sunburn to the very serious third-degree burn. Burns can cause tissue damage, depending on their severity. First-degree burns are characterized by minor blistering and pain. Second-degree burns are more serious, characterized by blistering, scarring and damaged hair follicles. Third-degree burns can lead to shock and are characterized by charred skin, severe muscle and tissue damage, and body fluid and electrolyte loss. Third-degree burns require immediate medical attention. Untreated burns can lead to serious infection.

Definition

Burns are defined as destruction of the skin or deeper tissues from extreme heat.

Symptoms

Symptoms include redness of skin, blistering and acute pain, depending on the severity of the burn.

Supplement support for burns

- ❧ Kyo-Green
- ❧ Vitamin C: 5000 mg three times daily
- ❧ Grapefruit seed extract spray to prevent infection
- ❧ Bach Rescue Remedy (see page 62)
- ❧ Cold aloe vera gel for first- and second-degree burns (store in refrigerator)

Medical treatment

Apply ice water immediately to take the heat out of the burn. For chemical burns, apply baking soda or apple cider vinegar in warm water compresses. Make sure that you stay hydrated with plenty of water. Have a whey protein smoothie to aid the healing process.

CALLUSES/CORNS

Calluses are usually found on the feet and hands. Corns can form on or between the toes. They can be hard or soft depending on their location. Causes include poor foot alignment, wearing improperly fitted shoes, an overly acid system from poor diet laden with fat, sugars and processed foods, and staph or strep infection.

Definition

Calluses are hardened, thickened areas of dead skin formed from keratin, externally caused by friction or pressure.

Symptoms

Symptoms include inflammation and pain in areas of either calluses or corns, which may ache and be tender to the touch.

Dietary considerations

Avoid fried, sugary and fatty foods. Eat fresh vegetables and fruits, and drink fresh fruit juices to detoxify and neutralize acidity.

Lifestyle choices

- ❧ Soak affected areas in sea salt or Epsom salts, and use a pumice stone to gently file the top layer. Afterwards, rub feet with warm almond oil, concentrating on the corn or callus.
- ❧ Make sure to wear shoes that fit properly and that do not cramp or pinch the toes or foot.
- ❧ Never use a sharp instrument of any kind to cut or shave the hardened areas away. To do so may cause infection. This is especially true for diabetics.

CANCER

Just hearing the word *cancer* seems to spark fear in the average person. Virtually all of us have been touched somehow by this dreaded disease. The good news is that while the cases of cancer are increasing, there is a rising group of cancer survivors because our knowledge about the disease has changed. Early detection has always been one factor in survival and proper treatment.

We now know that most cancers respond positively to diet improvement. By avoiding dead, de-mineralized, heavily processed foods, refined sugars, excessive caffeine, food dyes and sprayed foods (pesticides), which cancer cells thrive on, we can help our bodies rebuild healthy cells while "starving out" cancer cells.

Cancer attacks when the immune response is low, whether from overwork, emotional upheaval, poor diet or exposure to toxic substances. All of these factors change your body chemistry in a negative way, making it hard for your immune system to defend you from disease. Diet improvement will boost the immune system that has failed you by allowing cancer cells to form. You must create an environment in your body where cancer cannot flourish.

Knowledge is key to conquering the disease, especially learning to know the early detection signs listed below. I have included specifics for several kinds of cancer that are helpful in fighting the disease.

Definition

Cancer is a disease in which there is a dangerous, unrestrained growth of cells in an organ or body tissue.

Symptoms

Here are seven early detection signs:

1. Change in bowel or bladder habits, especially blood in the stool
2. Chronic indigestion, bloating, heartburn and difficulty swallowing
3. Unusual bleeding or discharge from the vagina
4. Lump or thickening of the breast or testicles
5. Chronic cough or constant hoarseness, bloody sputum
6. Changes or growth in warts or moles—dry, scaly skin patches that never heal, especially if they are inflamed or ulcerate
7. Unusual weight loss

CUT YOUR RISK FOR CANCER

Two fruits and three vegetables a day show promising anticancer results. (In this case, more is better!)

Reduce animal fat intake. (Toxins and pesticides are stored or lodged in animal fat.)

Limit red meat intake.

Boost your immune system. (Follow the guide in my book *90-Day Immune System Makeover*, published in 2000 by Siloam Press.)

Detoxify your body twice a year, in the spring and fall.

Take enzymes daily to digest, assimilate and eliminate properly.

Drink plenty of water, eight to ten glasses per day.

If you are on hormone therapy, use the lowest dose. Have blood or saliva levels run routinely to insure proper dosage.

CANCER, CERVICAL AND UTERINE

Women who are overweight, smoke, use estrogen replacement therapy, have never been pregnant or have given birth more than five times, or have a history of STD or abortion are at higher risk for cervical and uterine cancer.

Symptoms

Symptoms include a class 4 Pap smear (precancerous), unusual bleeding, discharge between menstrual periods, heavy painful periods and bleeding during intercourse.

Dietary considerations

Eliminate all dairy and meats from your diet, and add fresh fruits and vegetables, especially oranges and carrots. Add soy foods to your diet also.

Supplement support for cervical and uterine cancer

- Progesterone cream
- Green drinks daily
- Flax oil
- Royal jelly
- Ester C: 5,000–10,000 mg

CANCER, COLON AND COLORECTAL

Colon cancer begins as polyps on the colon walls.

Symptoms

Symptoms include blood in bowel movements, change in the shape of the stool to a thin, flattened appearance, persistent diarrhea changing to persistent constipation for no apparent reason and pain in the lower right abdomen. There is also unusual weight loss or fatigue.

Dietary considerations

Eat high-fiber foods and reduce intake of all meat. Add soy foods and plenty of tomatoes, fresh vegetables (dark greens and broccoli) and salads.

Eliminate refined sugars, pies, cakes and white flour.

Supplement support for colon and colorectal cancer

- Vitamin C: 3000 to 5000 mg daily
- Beta carotene: 100,000 IU
- Vitamin E: 800 IU with 200 mcg of selenium
- Flax oil
- Green tea: 1 to 3 cups daily
- Coenzyme Q_{10}: 100 mg two times daily
- Acidophilus capsules with meals
- Kyolic Garlic capsules: six to ten daily
- Reishi mushroom capsules
- Astragalus
- Shiitake mushroom capsules
- Daily green drink (Kyo-Green)

CANCER, KIDNEY AND BLADDER

People with a history of smoking, cystitis and polycystic kidney disease are at increased risk for kidney and bladder cancer.

Symptoms

Symptoms include blood in the urine with urination difficulties. It can also be accompanied by loin pain (lower part of back and sides between ribs and pelvis).

Dietary considerations

Increase water intake to eight to ten glasses daily and eat lots of carrots. Carrot juice is wonderful as well. Eat fresh fruits daily.

Supplement support for kidney and bladder cancer

- Garlic: eight to ten capsules daily
- Bio-K: liquid acidophilus
- Vitamin A: 40,000 IU
- Vitamin B_6: 250 mg
- Vitamin C: 3000–5000 mg
- Vitamin E: 400 IU
- Zinc: 50 mg
- Selenium: 200 mcg

CANCER, LIVER AND PANCREATIC

Early symptoms of liver and pancreatic cancer are weight loss and extreme tiredness.

Dietary considerations

Eat lots of broccoli, cabbage, tomatoes and watercress. Add soy foods to your diet. And eliminate alcohol!

Supplement support for liver and pancreatic cancer

- Chlorella
- Kyo-Green
- Flax oil
- Vitamin C: 5,000–10,000 mg
- Milk thistle
- Schizandra
- Dandelion
- Enzymedica's Purify
- Coenzyme Q_{10}: 200 mg daily
- Chromium picolinate: 200 mcg daily

Lifestyle choices

- Eliminate all alcohol consumption.
- Use coffee enemas.

Health Update　　**Coffee Enema: A Standard in Alternative Medicine**

Coffee enemas are used in natural medicine to help heal blood- and liver-related cancers. The caffeine in coffee stimulates the liver and gallbladder to remove toxins, produce necessary enzyme activity, open bile ducts and encourage peristaltic action.

Coffee enema formula: 1 cup regular coffee (strongly brewed) mixed with one quart water. (May be used prior to the liver flush. For details see page 223.)

Cancer, Lung

Lung cancer is the leading cause of cancer deaths worldwide.[29] Almost 90 percent of all lung cancer cases can be attributed to cigarette smoking.[30]

Symptoms

Symptoms include a persistent cough that continually worsens and is accompanied by chest pain; there may also be blood in the sputum and a sore throat or hoarseness. As the disease progresses, more intense chest pain along with weight loss, fever and unusual sweating will be experienced.

Dietary considerations

Reduce intake of all dairy foods and eat garlic and onions daily, along with shiitake mushrooms, broccoli and tomatoes. Eat a low-fat diet and add soy foods to your menu. Drink green tea daily.

Supplement support for lung cancer

- Germanium: 200 mg
- Vitamin E: 1000 IU

* Vitamin C: 3000–5000 mg (critical!)
* B complex: 150 mg
* Beta carotene: 100,000 IU

Lifestyle choices
  Stop smoking!

CANCER, OVARIAN

Women who are more at risk are those who never had children, are post-menopausal, eat a high-fat diet, take long-term estrogen replacement therapy or use talcum powder.

Symptoms
  Symptoms include bloating, tiredness and abdominal discomfort.

Dietary considerations
  Eat lots of fresh fruit and vegetables, add soy foods to your diet and avoid fried foods and eggs.

Supplement support for ovarian cancer

* Beta carotene: 150,000 IU
* Milk thistle
* Garlic: eight to ten capsules
* Progesterone cream
* Ester C: 5,000–10,000 mg
* Vitamin E: 800 IU daily
* Selenium: 200 mcg
* Daily green drink
* Shark cartilage
* Bovine tracheal cartilage
* Royal jelly

Health Update — No-Nos for Ovarian Cancer Risk

Women who use talcum powder in the vaginal area after bathing increase their risk of ovarian cancer by 60 percent. Women using powder deodorant sprays for the vaginal area have a 90 percent increased risk. Avoid these products![31]

CANCER, PROSTATE AND TESTICULAR

Because prostate and testicular cancers are the most common cancers in males, I recommend that you have a PSA (prostate specific antigen) test yearly.[32]

Symptoms

Symptoms include frequent urination, lump in the testicles or prostate, back pain and difficulty starting and stopping urination.

Dietary considerations

Eliminate caffeine from your diet, and add fiber, tomatoes (better when cooked), broccoli, cauliflower, whole grains and soybeans. Avoid all animal fats as well.

Supplement support for prostate and testicular cancer

- Green tea daily
- Beta carotene: 100,000 IU
- Royal jelly
- Saw palmetto
- Pygeum
- Pumpkinseed oil
- Vitamin C: 10,000 mg
- Glutathione: 100 mg daily
- Vitamin E: 400 IU
- Coenzyme Q_{10}: 200 mg daily
- Evening primrose oil

WARNING: Do not take DHEA if you have prostate cancer. It may stimulate the cancer!

ACS Guidelines for Early Detection of Cancer

Cervical

Women who are or have been sexually active or have reached eighteen years of age should have a Pap test and pelvic exam every year; after three or more consecutive satisfactory normal annual exams, the Pap test may be performed less frequently at the discretion of the physician.

Breast

Women age forty and older should have an annual mammogram and an annual clinical breast exam by their healthcare professional, and they should do a monthly breast self-exam. The clinical breast exam should be done a short time before the mammogram. Women ages twenty to thirty-nine should have a clinical breast exam every three years and should do monthly breast self-exams.

Prostate

Men age fifty and older should have both a digital rectal exam and the prostate-specific antigen (PSA) test every year.

Colorectal

Men and women age fifty and older should have a sigmoidoscopy every three to five years and a fecal occult blood test every year.[33]

CANCER, STOMACH AND ESOPHAGEAL

Stomach and esophageal cancer are directly linked to a high-fat, low-fiber diet, to H. pylori (helicobacter pylori is a bacterium that infects the stomach) and to smoking.

Symptoms

Symptoms include gastritis, pain after eating, chronic indigestion and pernicious anemia.

Dietary considerations

You should include the following in your diet: fresh vegetables, whole wheat, broccoli, onions, garlic, cabbage, avocados, soy, grapefruit and tomatoes.

Supplement support for stomach and esophageal cancer

- Glutathione: 100 mg daily
- Kyolic Garlic capsules: six to eight daily
- Green tea
- Coenzyme Q_{10}: 200 mg daily
- Beta carotene
- Vitamin C
- Vitamin E
- Bio-K: liquid acidophilus followed by Kyo-Dophilus

Lifestyle choices

- Eat small meals only.
- Have a green drink daily (Kyo-Green).
- Use Enzymedica's Purify for body cleansing.
- Get professional help to stop smoking.

CANDIDIASIS/CANDIDA

Candida is a stress-related condition marked by a seriously compromised immune response. *Candida albicans* normally lives harmlessly in our gastrointestinal tracts and the genito-urinary areas of our body. If our immune response is reduced, as mine was from repeated courses of antibiotics, by a high-sugar diet and lack of rest and relaxation, candida then multiplies too quickly, resulting in major health problems. These yeast colonies establish a foothold and flourish throughout the body, releasing toxins into the bloodstream. The toxins that are released trigger many symptoms, including those listed below.

Definition

Candida can be defined as infection of the skin or mucous membrane with any species of candida, but chiefly *candida albicans,* usually localized in the skin, nails, mouth, vagina, vulva, bronchi or lungs, but it may also infect the bloodstream.

Symptoms

Symptoms include constipation, diarrhea, colitis, bloating, muscle and joint pain, clogged sinuses, vaginitis, kidney and bladder infections, memory loss and mood swings, adrenal problems, low blood sugar, thyroid problems, hormonal imbalances, severe itching, prostatitis, dizziness, foggy thinking, extreme fatigue, loss of memory, weight gain, weight loss, vaginal yeast infections, anxiety and depression, and as many as a hundred other symptoms.

CANDIDA: A PLAN OF ATTACK

- Kill the yeast through diet change and supplement support.

- Avoid antibiotics unless absolutely necessary. There are natural antibiotic alternatives.

- Detoxify the body to cleanse the dead yeast from the body.

- Use enzyme therapy to strengthen the digestive system in order to assimilate nutrients. Strengthen the liver and kidneys. "Re-plant" healthy bowel flora with friendly bacteria.

- Rebuild immunity. Follow my *90-Day Immune System Makeover* (Siloam Press, 2000).

- Additional reading: *The Fungus Link* by Dr. Doug Kaufman (Mediatrician Pub., 2001)

Dietary considerations

The classic candida diet permits dense protein foods, such as chicken and fish, and as many vegetables as you can eat. Some people can use whole grains, while others cannot. Caffeine and alcohol should be avoided, as should foods made from flour: breads, pastas, tortillas, cakes, cookies, etc. Eliminate all sugar and sugar-containing foods. Read food labels carefully, as thousands of packaged foods contain sucrose, dextrose, glucose, fructose, corn syrup, maple syrup, honey, molasses, barley malt, rice syrup, etc. If sweetening is required, use Stevia.

Avoid foods that contain vinegar (mustard, mayonnaise, etc.), fermented foods (cheese, sauerkraut, soy sauce, etc.) and processed meats, especially hot dogs, sausages, bacon, etc.

Try to drink only filtered or bottled water as tap water contains chlorine, which will further reduce the body's populations of friendly flora.

If you are a strict vegetarian, it is difficult to obtain enough complete protein without overloading on grains and beans. Eating a wide variety of vegetables, at the same time, can help counter this problem, as can supplements like spirulina and chlorella. Books with recipes for the candida diet can be invaluable.

While the candida diet is rigid, it is necessary. As you begin to get yeast under control, you may be able to increase the levels of grains you eat and to add some fruits. If you do, be careful to monitor the way you feel, and at the first sign of recurring discomforts, return to the strict diet.

Supplement support for candida

- ❦ Candex: four capsules per day until the discomfort is under control (See Health Update below.)
- ❦ Probiotic supplements lactobacillus acidophilus and lactobacillus bifidus: one capsule with a meal twice daily (See explanation on page 41.)
- ❦ Use natural antibiotics (See page 42.)

Health Update   **Breakthrough in Candida Management**

Candex is a natural yeast management by Pure Essence Labs (888-254-8000). Each capsule of Candex contains about 52,000 units of cellulase digesting activity.

With the advent of digestive enzymes, a new tool against candida has emerged. Since candida's cell wall is made largely of cellulose, cellulase enzymes break it down. As this occurs, the yeast dies.

Cellulase enzymes do not harm the liver and are safe in every way. Further, because candida cannot change the structure of its cell wall, it cannot become immune to these enzymes. Finally, because the enzymes do not cause the yeast to release toxins, you'll begin to feel better almost immediately and with no healing crisis (die-off reaction) whatever.

Most people respond best to about 200,000 CU's of cellulase per day. Candex is the only product that is commonly available (through health food store, natural health practitioners and physicians) that provides these levels.

CAUTION: While some people say that after using Candex they have been able to reintroduce wider varieties of foods without incident, others report a rapid recurrence of discomforts when they do this.

CHOLESTEROL—HIGH

Americans have been educated that they need to make sure their cholesterol levels are not too high because high cholesterol is considered a major factor in the development of heart disease. That is only part of the truth. Actually, cholesterol itself is not bad; it is a necessary fat made up of LDL, HDL and several other components.

HDL is "good cholesterol," keeping molecules from sticking to the sides of the arteries. LDL is the "bad cholesterol" that has sticky properties and can slow down the flow of blood to the heart, causing a heart attack and death.

Triglycerides are sugar-related blood fats that travel through the bloodstream along with HDL and LDL. High triglycerides also cause blood cells to stick together, increasing the risk of heart attack.

Definition

High cholesterol can be defined as an excessive amount in the blood of the organic compound present in animal fats and also manufactured by the human body.

Symptoms

Symptoms include cold hands and feet, difficulty breathing, heart palpitations, dizziness, high blood pressure, poor circulation and fatigue.

Causes

High stress levels can cause an overproduction of adrenaline. Most hormones, including adrenaline, are manufactured from cholesterol. Therefore, when more adrenaline is needed, more cholesterol is manufactured.

Genetic predisposition through heredity also causes high cholesterol.

Overconsumption of foods that are high in saturated fats and cholesterol, like butter, eggs, cheese, heavy cream and fatty meats, is a lifestyle cause.

Diuretics can raise cholesterol by causing essential minerals to be excreted. Mineral loss causes stress on the nervous system, leading to an increased need for adrenaline.

Levels of cholesterol will rise in women who have difficulty converting cholesterol to estrogen and progesterone.

Health Update	Ideal Cholesterol Levels

Ideal levels are as follows:

Triglyceride levels: 170–200 mg/dl
Cholesterol: 140–165 mg/dl
LDL: 30–50 mg/dl
HDL: 80–90 mg/dl

NOTE: Over 244 mg/dl means increased heart attack risk.

Dietary considerations

Avoid or limit red meat, fried foods, full-fat dairy foods, sugary and refined foods. Add to your diet the following: garlic, high-fiber foods, fruits and vegetables, soy foods, olive oil, yogurt and beans. Have a glass of red wine with dinner to reduce stress.

Supplement support for high cholesterol

- Red yeast rice
- Coenzyme Q$_{10}$: 60–100 mg daily
- Grapeseed PCOs: 100 mg daily
- Flax oil
- Kyolic Garlic capsules
- Chromium picolinate: 200 mcg daily
- Guggul lipid
- Green tea
- Milk thistle
- Flush-free niacin
- Carnitine: 1000 mg daily
- Lecithin: 2 tablespoons of granules daily
- Choline
- Inositol

Lifestyle choices

- Exercise regularly; take a walk daily.
- Reduce body weight.
- Stop smoking.
- Reduce stress.
- Have regular massage therapy to release tension.

Health Update   Policosanol

Policosanol, a natural approach to reducing cardiovascular disease, is an anti-cholesterol dietary supplement that works as well as statin drugs. Policosanol is made from sugar cane and has been shown to lower cholesterol without life-threatening side effects.

Policosanol...

- Elevates HDL better than most statin drugs.
- Inhibits the formation of lesion in arteries.
- Keeps LDL from oxidizing.
- Enhances the benefits of exercise and reduces complications in people with artery diseases.
- Reduces thromboxane, which promotes inflammation.

The main ingredient in policosanol is octacosanol, an alcohol found in the waxy film that plants have over their leaves and fruit. The rinds of citrus fruits and wheat germ oil both contain octacosanol.

NOTE: Policosanol should only be taken by people who have high-serum cholesterol levels. Recommended dose is 5 milligrams to 20 milligrams daily. The average person uses 10 milligrams daily.[34]

CORONARY HEART DISEASE (CHD) RISK FACTORS

Family history of premature heart disease (parent or sibling with CHD before age 55)

Male over 45

Female after menopause

Current cigarette smoker

High blood pressure (above 140/90)

High blood sugar level (diabetes)

Low HDL-cholesterol (<35 mg/dl): If HDL-cholesterol is >60 mg/dl, subtract one risk factor

Inactivity and lack of exercise

High-stress environment

Overweight

LDL-TARGET LEVELS

To determine what your LDL should be, count the risk factors that you marked above and use the guide below:

Without CHD and fewer than two risk factors: LDL should be <160 mg/dL.

Without CHD and two or more risk factors: LDL should be <130 mg/dL.

With CHD your target should be <100 mg/dL.

CHRONIC FATIGUE SYNDROME

This condition has a variety of causes. Researchers have found that a number of viruses are actually involved, including Epstein-Barr virus, Cytomegalo virus and herpes simplex. Parasites and candida albicans are often found as part of the clinical picture as well. Exhausted adrenal glands and lowered immunity set the stage for this medically incurable viral condition.

Most victims are women usually between the ages of twenty-four and forty-five who share the following profile: overachiever, outgoing, A-type personality, independent and self-reliant. This profiles a person with high-stress levels and lowered adrenal health.[35] Natural therapies focus on building the adrenal health, eliminating candida and parasites and boosting immune function.

Definition

Chronic fatigue syndrome is a health disorder characterized by feelings of debilitation and lack of energy.

Symptoms

Symptoms for the first stage of chronic fatigue include debilitating fatigue, which does not resolve with bed rest for at least six months, low-grade fever, sore throat, muscle weakness, gastrointestinal problems and sore lymph nodes.

Symptoms for the second stage include ringing in the ears, depression, irritability, allergies, vertigo, sharp muscle aches and low blood sugar—hypoglycemia.

Third-stage symptoms include night sweats, frequent infections, weight loss, loss of appetite, extreme fatigue, fainting, extremely low immunity, heart palpitations and nervous system disorders.

Dietary considerations

Eat fresh whole foods: brown rice, high fiber, yogurt, dark leafy vegetables, prunes, wheat germ, vegetable juices, garlic and onions. Avoid refined sugars, alcohol, dairy and wheat.

Supplement support for chronic fatigue syndrome

- Digestive plant enzymes
- B complex
- Magnesium chloride: 800 mg
- Royal jelly
- Reishi mushroom capsules
- Carnitine: 2000 mg daily
- Adrenal Glandular
- Ester C: 3000–5000 mg
- Daily green drink
- Olive leaf extract
- Grapefruit seed extract
- Candex: for yeast eradication
- Milk thistle extract
- Bio K: acidophilus
- Astragalus
- Coenzyme Q_{10}: 100 mg daily

Lifestyle choices

- Have a massage at least three times monthly.
- Manage stress levels.
- Begin a walking program.
- Spend fifteen minutes in morning sunlight.

Health Update	Overlooked Causes of Chronic Fatigue

Overactive thyroid	Hormonal problems
Underactive thyroid	Food allergies
Adrenal insufficiency	Environmental toxins
Diabetes	Hypoglycemia

A HIDDEN CAUSE OF FATIGUE

If you suffer from fatigue, you may have an iodine deficiency. A lack of iodine can impair your thyroid function. And a sluggish thyroid can leave you feeling tired and weak.

Fortunately, there's an excellent test you can do at home to check your iodine levels. Simply take a Q-tip, dip it into a 2 percent tincture of iodine (available at any drugstore or supermarket) and paint a two-inch square on your thigh or belly. This will leave a yellowish stain that should disappear in about twenty-four hours if your iodine levels are normal.

If the stain disappears in less than twenty-four hours, it means your body is deficient in iodine and has thirstily sucked it up. If that's the case, keep applying the iodine every day at different sites, until the stain lasts a full twenty-four hours.

Not only will you have diagnosed your iodine deficiency, but you will have treated that deficiency and improved your thyroid function!

CIRCULATION PROBLEMS

Circulation problems can signal a serious problem. High blood pressure, varicose veins, phlebitis, arteriosclerosis and heart disease are all associated with poor or sluggish circulation. Causes include lack of exercise, low-fiber diet, constipation, internal toxicity, stress and high cholesterol—all causing plaque buildup on arterial walls.

Definition
Circulation problems are defined as sluggish blood flow leading to cardio-vascular problems.

Symptoms
Symptoms include poor memory, cold hands and feet, headaches, ringing in the ears, hearing loss, shortness of breath, dizziness, leg cramps, varicose veins, high cholesterol, high triglycerides and swollen ankles.

Dietary considerations

Eat a diet that is high in fiber, and, if necessary, take a fiber supplement daily to keep your colon clear. Avoid large or heavy meals, and take digestive enzymes with your meal. Drink six to eight glasses of water daily. Eat plenty of citrus fruits and juices for strong veins and tissue walls. Limit your intake of salt, caffeine, sugar, red meat and fatty, fried foods. Add garlic to your recipes. Drink green tea daily.

Supplement support for circulation problems

- Liquid chlorophyll
- Carnitine: 500 mg
- Vitamin E: 400 IU
- Quercetin: 500 mg twice daily
- Bromelain: 500 mg twice daily
- Flax oil
- Coenzyme Q_{10}: 60 mg daily
- Garlic (Kyolic capsules)
- Lecithin granules or capsules
- Ester C: 3,000 mg
- Gingko biloba
- Ginger tea
- Butcher's broom
- PCOs (grapeseed extract): 100 mg daily

Lifestyle choices

- Have weekly massages until condition improves, then monthly.
- Start a walking program to stimulate circulation.
- Practice dry skin brushing before showering.
- Apply ginger packs to kidney.
- Try swimming, which is excellent for circulation.

COLDS

The common cold...annoying? Yes. But in natural medicine, a cold is thought of as your body's attempt to cleanse itself of toxins, wastes, bacteria and mucus that have built up to a point where the immune system is overwhelmed. The healing approach of natural medicine for this condition is to work the body instead of trying to suppress symptoms with over-the-counter cold medications.

Definition

A cold is defined as a viral infection of the upper respiratory tract.

Symptoms

Symptoms include sore throat, headache, fever, head congestion, sneezing and aches and pains.

Dietary considerations

Enjoy grandma's homemade chicken soup. Eliminate dairy products, sugar and fried foods to increase mucus release. Drink plenty of fluids, including water with lemon, green drink and diluted fruit juices. Eat lightly, with plenty of steamed vegetables and fresh fruits.

Supplement support for the common cold

- Vitamin C: 3000 mg
- Grapefruit seed extract capsules
- Echinacea
- Ginger compress on chest
- White flower oil on throat area, neck and chest
- NutriBiotic Nasal Spray
- NAC (N-acetyl cysteine)
- Kyolic Garlic: six capsules daily
- Goldenseal
- Beta glucan

Lifestyle choices

REST! Allow yourself some down time to recover completely. After the acute phase passes, take short daily walks to stimulate circulation.

COLITIS

Most colitis sufferers are between the ages of twenty and forty with stressful occupations or lifestyles, with females being slightly more prone to colitis than males.[36] Natural therapies are very effective and can reduce the need for harsh medications. Most cases are related to food allergies, which in turn cause an inflamed colon. Typically, cheese, corn, wheat and eggs are the most common colitis triggers. Diet change is imperative in relieving and healing colitis. The following recommendations have been used with great success.

Definition

Colitis is an inflammation of the large intestine, accompanied by diarrhea, constipation and cramping.

Symptoms

Symptoms include pain, gas, bloody diarrhea, ulcers in the colon lining and hard stools.

Causes

Colitis may be caused by emotional stress, depression and anxiety, lack of fiber, food allergies, candida yeast involvement, vitamin K deficiency, too many antibiotics, excess sugar and refined foods in the diet.

Dietary considerations

Clean up your diet. Avoid coffee, caffeine, nuts, dairy and citrus foods. Cut out sugar, wheat and spicy foods. Eat yogurt every day, and drink plenty of water daily, at least six to eight glasses. Make one glass a green drink. Make oatmeal, brown rice, steamed veggies, green salads and fresh fruits, especially apples, a part of your diet. Eat smaller meals. It is easier for you to digest and assimilate your food.

Supplement support for colitis

- ❦ Take milk thistle extract for liver health.
- ❦ Have a cup of chamomile tea before bed, sweetened with Stevia.
- ❦ Use Bio-K probiotic culture liquid for intestinal rebalancing and rebuilding.
- ❦ Calm the body with kava, valerian or passionflower tea before bed.
- ❦ For cramping, try cramp bark capsules.
- ❦ Take glucosamine sulfate, 500 mg daily, for mucous membrane rebuilding.
- ❦ Use Siberian ginseng to fortify the body during times of stress.
- ❦ Take royal jelly for adrenal gland health.

Health Update   Natural Help for IBS

One in five adults suffers from the chronic and debilitating distress of irritable bowel syndrome.[37] The symptoms include severe bloating, gas, constipation, diarrhea and cramping.

Calm Colon is an effective irritable bowel syndrome formula, clinically proven for internal bowel support. Calm Colon was proven effective in double-blind placebo-controlled clinical trials. Take one capsule, three times daily. (You can order Calm Colon by calling 800-669-2256.)

IBS can also be controlled with two herbs:

- ❦ Peppermint relaxes the smooth muscle surrounding the large intestine, curbing spasms. During flare-ups take one or two enteric-coated peppermint oil capsules three times daily between meals.

- ❦ St. John's wort acts as a mild tranquilizer and antidepressant, thereby relieving emotional stress. Take one capsule two times daily with meals.[38]

COLON HEALTH

In natural medicine, it is generally agreed that disease begins in the colon. Poor elimination contributes to most health conditions. As a personal insurance policy against internal toxicity, make sure to eat a diet that is high in fiber, low in animal fat and that includes plenty of fresh fruits and vegetables. These dietary considerations will have a two-pronged effect. First, it will prevent improper elimination. Second, it will prevent or help to heal the diseases that elimination problems cause.

Unless you eliminate properly, unreleased wastes can be a breeding ground for parasitic infections. Intestinal parasites feed on fermented, rancid and over-accumulated amounts of food that remain in the intestinal tract. This can lead to lowered immunity, tissue degeneration, poor circulation and sluggish organ and glandular function. The first step in boosting colon health is to cleanse the colon.

There are obvious symptoms of an unhealthy digestive tract: poor digestion, bad breath, lower backache, fatigue, poor skin, body odor, gas and stomach bloating, to name a few. Internal toxicity has several causes: poor diet with a lack of live foods (fresh fruit and vegetables), lack of proper enzyme activity, constipation and a lack of water to flush toxins and speed up the digestive and eliminative process. Stress also hinders proper digestion, absorption and elimination.

Overuse of antibiotics has a damaging effect on the intestinal tract as well. Antibiotic therapy removes healthy and unhealthy bacteria in the colon. This causes yeast overgrowth, digestive problems and elimination problems. Overeating and eating late at night inhibit cleansing and restorative processes and puts too much stress on the digestive system.

Dietary considerations

Avoid sugar, animal fats, fried foods and dairy foods. Drink six to eight glasses of water daily; add fresh lemon to enhance cleansing effect. Add fiber foods to improve transit time, which should be ten to twelve hours. About 40 grams of fiber daily is recommended.

Supplement support for colon health

- Nature's Secret Ultimate Cleanse

After cleansing the colon:

- Magnesium: 400 mg daily
- Bio-K or Kyo-Dophilus to replenish intestinal tract with healthy bowel flora
- Digestive enzyme with every meal
- Milk thistle extract for liver function
- Colon Clenz by Natural Balance, Inc., for occasional bowel sluggishness
- Nature's Secret Ultimate Oil to prevent constipation

Lifestyle choices

Begin a walking program to stimulate circulation. Exercise stimulates the circulatory and lymphatic system. It raises metabolic efficiency and enhances the body's natural cleansing ability. Also, consider colonic irrigations given by a colonic therapist. To relieve stress, you can have a massage.

CONGESTIVE HEART FAILURE

The discussion of heart attack and other related heart issues in this book will give you the information you need regarding congestive heart failure.

Definition
Congestive heart failure is a condition in which the heart is unable to pump blood efficiently.

Symptoms
Symptoms include dizziness and shortness of breath after exertion, nausea, gas, swollen ankles and feet, and fluid in the lungs.

SEE HEART ATTACK AND RELATED HEART CONDITIONS.

CONSTIPATION

As we have mentioned, natural medicine holds that disease and death begin in the colon. Old, impacted waste material often reabsorbs into the body and nearby organs and sets the stage for diseases, viruses, parasites and candida. The causes of constipation are varied and include stress, hypothyroidism, low-fiber diet, poor diet with too much sugar, fast foods, processed foods, allergy to dairy products, prescription drugs and lack of exercise. If you are not having a bowel movement at least once a day, then technically you are constipated and your bowels are sluggish. Bowel transit time should be twelve hours. Many Americans have only three bowel movements a week.

Definition
Constipation is defined as infrequent and/or uncomfortable bowel movements.

Symptoms
Symptoms include irritability, headache, fatigue, nausea, flatulence, gas, body odor, bad breath and poor skin tone.

Dietary considerations
Drink plenty of water, six to eight glasses daily. You should avoid high-fat, sugary and fried foods along with dairy foods because they hamper your body's efforts to rid itself of wastes. Remember, your body loves fiber. I call fiber your body's "little house cleaner." It helps to sweep all of the toxins and wastes through your intestines in record time. The following chart will help you decide if you need to increase your fiber intake.

> **Health Update**   Optimal Elimination Index

The following guidelines will insure that your elimination is optimal:

- ❦ There should be almost no gas or flatulence.
- ❦ The stool should be almost odorless, which means transit time is good.
- ❦ The stool should be light enough to float, indicating adequate fiber intake.
- ❦ The bowel movement should be effortless, daily and regular.

If you are not on track, simply add a fiber supplement until you achieve the desired results. By using this guide, you will be able to make your constipation a thing of the past. Remember to drink plenty of water when adding fiber to the diet!

Supplement support for constipation

- ❦ Acidophilus liquid at first, then switch to capsules
- ❦ Magnesium: 400–800 mg daily
- ❦ Cascara sagrada, a natural laxative
- ❦ Senna leaf, a natural laxative
- ❦ Flax oil
- ❦ Nature's Secret Ultimate Cleanse to detoxify
- ❦ Kyolic Garlic liquid
- ❦ Digestive plant enzymes
- ❦ Daily green drink
- ❦ Peppermint tea
- ❦ Ginger tea

Lifestyle choices

Take a brisk daily walk to promote regularity. (See Bowel Function Test in Part Four.)

CROHN'S DISEASE—REGIONAL ENTERITIS

This painful autoimmune disease affects over two million Americans today, and the numbers are rising.[39] This is mostly because so many people consistently eat diets that are low in fiber and too much refined sugar and suffer from food allergies, yeast overgrowth and emotional stress.

Definition

Crohn's disease is a chronic inflammation of the digestive tract, accompanied by painful ulcers that form in one or more sections.

Symptoms

Symptoms include painful ulcers that form in one or more sections of the gastrointestinal tract, diarrhea, abdominal pain, low-grade fever, weight loss, depression, anemia, wheat sensitivity, gas, inflammation and soreness.

Immune system function declines due to malnutrition.

Dietary considerations

Gradually increase your fiber intake until you are eating a substantially high-fiber diet, except during flare-ups of the disease. Drink eight to ten glasses of spring water daily. Consume fresh juices and vegetables daily (grape, carrot, apple and pineapple are especially therapeutic). Avoid red and fatty meats as well as dairy and fried foods. Eliminate seeds, popcorn and nuts.

Supplement support for Crohn's disease

- Magnesium: 400–800 mg daily
- Bio-K Liquid Acidophilus during flare-ups, then Kyo-Dophilus capsules
- Glutamine: 500 mg
- Vitamin C
- Royal jelly
- Quercetin
- Kyolic Garlic capsules: six daily
- Green tea
- Flax oil
- Daily green drink
- Peppermint tea sweetened with Stevia

Lifestyle choices

- Reduce stress.
- Have regular massages.
- Practice deep breathing.
- Eat early, eat less, but eat often.

CYSTITIS

Cystitis is very common in women. As a matter of fact, bladder infections are the most frequent reason a woman seeks medical attention.[40] You should begin treating this condition at the first sign of infection.

Definition

Cystitis is inflammation of the bladder.

Symptoms

Symptoms include a frequent urge and desire to empty the bladder along with painful urination; the urine may appear cloudy and have a strong smell.

Common causes

Causes of cystitis include overuse of antibiotics, *E. coli* that migrates up the urethra, stress, kidney malfunction, food allergens, lack of water, poor elimination and a need for detoxification. The following protocol may be used for healing as well as for a preventative maintenance program.

Dietary considerations

Follow an improved eating plan that is free of yeast, sugar and dairy. Drink six to eight glasses of unsweetened cranberry juice or take cranberry concentrate gel capsules as directed. In addition, drink plenty of water. Eat watermelon or drink watermelon juice. Eliminate caffeine, chocolate, red meat, sugary foods, soft drinks and dairy foods.

Supplement support for cystitis

- Grapefruit seed extract capsules
- Kyolic Garlic capsules daily if the problem is chronic
- A liquid probiotic supplement like Bio-K daily
- Daily green drink (Kyo-Green by Wakunaga)

CYSTS AND POLYPS

Many times toxicity or infection can contribute to the occurrence of cysts and polyps. Other causes include poor diet with mucus- or acid-promoting foods, poor assimilation and improper digestion of fats.

Definition

Cysts are closed pockets of tissue, which can be filled with air, pus or other material.

Symptoms

Symptoms may vary depending on the location of the cyst or polyp. A cyst is characterized by a lump or bulge under the skin that is usually moveable. In the case of vaginal cysts and cervical, colon, bladder or rectal polyps, there is often bleeding vaginally, rectally or in the urine. The good news is that cysts and polyps are benign. However, some (usually colon polyps) can lead to cancer without proper treatment.

Dietary considerations

Eliminate all fried foods, animal fats, chocolate, margarine, caffeine, dairy and white flour. Eat fresh fruits to help detoxify your system. Drink eight to ten glasses of water daily to flush toxins.

Supplement support for cysts and polyps

- Coenzyme Q_{10}: 100 mg daily
- Milk thistle liquid extract
- Echinacea extract
- Pau d'arco tea sweetened with Stevia
- Calcium: 1500 mg daily
- Carlson's ACES + Zinc
- Ester C: 3000 mg daily
- Flax oil
- Cayenne capsules

Lifestyle choices
Internally, use Nature's Secret Ultimate Cleanse to cleanse the blood, liver, colon and kidneys. For external growths, apply tea tree oil. Scrub the skin with loofah to keep pores unclogged during detoxification.

DANDRUFF

Dandruff can be a source of embarrassment. In our society, it seems to be socially unacceptable to be seen with telltale white flakes of dandruff on our shoulders. Many television commercials promote special shampoos or potions to control this condition, but it can be naturally overcome with better diet and supplementation. The two main types of dandruff, seborrheic and pityriasis (simple dandruff), respond well to diet improvement.

Definition
Dandruff is a skin condition generally of the scalp, characterized by dry or greasy white scales, with or without reddening of the skin.

Symptoms
Symptoms of dandruff include scaling flakes on the scalp, eyebrows and face (occasionally), which can be caused by allergy or essential fatty acid deficiency.

Dietary considerations
Limit sugars and animal fats. Eat yogurt or take acidophilus liquid daily. Avoid chocolate, dairy, nuts and shellfish. Eat eggs, wheat germ, fish (salmon), onions, lettuce, fresh fruit and vegetables.

Supplement support for dandruff
The following supplements may be considered scalp food:

- Zinc picolinate: 50 mg two times daily
- Biotin: 600 mcg daily
- B complex
- PABA: 1000 mg daily
- Essential fatty acids: Nature's Secret Ultimate Oil or NOW 3-6-9
- Carlson ACES

Health Update   Help for Hair

Rinse hair with apple cider vinegar every other day. Also, use a small amount of tea tree oil or a few drops of grapefruit seed extract added to your shampoo daily. You may alternate the two for best results.

Lifestyle choices
Exercise regularly, and massage your head each day to stimulate circulation.

DENTAL PROBLEMS: TMJ, PERIODONTAL DISEASE, TOOTHACHES AND MORE

Ten million people suffer from TMJ (temporomandibular joint syndrome).[41] About 90 percent of all Americans have some form of gum disease or tooth decay, including half of the population over the age of thirty-five.[42] A toothache can cause the worst kind of pain. The best offense is defense when it comes to your dental health.

Proper oral hygiene is essential, which includes proper brushing and flossing. I recommend using HydroFloss and the Dental Herb Company's natural herbal mouth rinse. (Ask your dentist about these two products.)

Lowered immunity seems to play a part in the development of periodontal disease. Unfortunately, many children are showing signs of gum disease. Stress management and immune enhancement are imperative in the fight against this progressive disorder. Periodontal disease often coexists with cardiovascular problems.

Questions have been raised about the safety of mercury amalgam fillings. Many people are in fact sensitive to mercury fillings. However, removal can stir up vapor, making your sensitivity worse. After removal, a detoxification program is essential to cleanse the mercury from your blood stream. Work with your dentist gradually as you replace your mercury fillings with composite (white) or porcelain inlays.

Definition

Dental problems include toothaches, bruxism (teeth-grinding), decay, TMJ and periodontal disease.

Symptoms

In all dental difficulties the two main symptoms are pain and sensitivity; in the case of bruxism there is also the grinding of the teeth.

AMALGAM REMOVAL DETOX PROTOCOL

Begin this protocol two weeks prior to first removal appointment, and continue for two or three months after the last amalgam removal appointment. These products are available at your health food store.

- Chlorella or Kyo-Green: Chlorella's cell wall binds to heavy metals like mercury and accelerates their removal from the body. I recommend that chlorella or Kyo-Green be taken indefinitely.
- Garlic: This cleansing herb enhances the effectiveness of chlorella.
- ACES Antioxidants: These supplements help protect cell membranes from free-radical damage.

    ❖ Ester C powder: Take 2 heaping teaspoons a day with or without food on the day before, the day of and the day after removal. Decrease dose if you experience diarrhea.

    ❖ Multivitamin and mineral: This supplement will replace lost minerals and vitamins.

    ❖ Cysteine: This is a chelator of heavy metals. Take as directed by manufacturer.

    ❖ Drink plenty of water.

Dietary considerations

Eat fresh fruits and vegetables to clean teeth. Fill your diet with foods such as apples, broccoli, cauliflower, celery, carrots, peppers, nuts and seeds. Eat plenty of healthy salads. Drink green tea to help prevent plaque formation. Use Stevia to sweeten as it is also antibacterial. Enjoy strawberry smoothies; strawberries also help prevent the formation of plaque.

Avoid or reduce sugars, fats, dairy products and candy to minimize the film on teeth that contributes to tooth decay.

Supplement support for dental problems

Special support for TMJ:

    ❖ Dr. Janet's Glucosamine Cream (¼ teaspoon to painful area as needed)

    ❖ B complex

    ❖ DLPA

    ❖ Anxiety Control 24 (patented formula)

    ❖ Coenzyme Q_{10}: 100 mg daily

    ❖ L–theanine

Special support for bruxism:

    ❖ Calcium

    ❖ Magnesium chloride

    ❖ Anxiety Control 24

Special support for general oral health:

    ❖ Coenzyme Q_{10}

    ❖ Ester C

    ❖ Omega-3 fatty acids

    ❖ Liquid chlorophyll (prepare a green drink before and after amalgam removal)

    ❖ Multivitamin

Lifestyle choices

    ❖ Have regular dental checkups!

    ❧   Brush your teeth twice daily (two minutes each time).

    ❧   Use natural toothpaste, such as Tom's of Maine or from Dental Herb Company.

    ❧   Use Natural Tooth and Gum Tonic from Dental Herb Company.

NOTE: If you suspect mercury toxicity, have a hair analysis performed since mercury does not show up in urine or blood samples.

DEPRESSION

Depression has risen to epidemic proportions in this country. More than 1.5 million people are being treated for it, and 30 million more can expect to suffer from it sometime in their lives.[43] Our emotions play a key role in this devastating condition, which leads to physical depletion. Women seem to be more susceptible to depression than men, perhaps because women are more overtly "emotional" or because there is perhaps a female reproductive hormone connection.

The underlying origins for depression are usually bottled-up anger or aggression turned inward, great emotional loss and the inability to express grief. Depression can also be the result of negative emotional behavior, often learned in childhood, in an attempt to control relationships. Some cases of depression are also drug-induced because prescription drugs create nutrient deficiencies.

Definition

Depression is a disorder characterized by a pervasive depressed mood, pessimistic thoughts and feelings of despair and hopelessness, accompanied by a loss of interest in otherwise pleasurable activities and changes in eating and sleeping habits.

Symptoms

Symptoms of depression include fatigue, headaches, loss of interest in pleasurable things, weight loss or weight gain, lethargy, heart palpitations and inability to concentrate.

Causes

Besides the emotional difficulties mentioned above, depression can be a result of prolonged stress, which causes a deficiency of amino acids, resulting in a biochemical imbalance. Other nutritional deficiencies, nervous tension, poor diet, mononucleosis, thyroid disorders, allergies and serious physical disorders can also cause depression.

Depression can definitely be connected to brain depletion. When certain nutrients are not supplied to the brain, a negative set of emotions can occur that affect our ability to cope with stressful situations that we confront each day. Scientific studies are showing that by taking specific amino acids to restore the brain, depression can be alleviated.[44]

Dietary considerations

Nutrition is crucial in the treatment of depression and is the key to your brain's behavior. Eat foods that are rich in calcium, magnesium and B vitamins. Eat foods that contain tryptophan, like turkey, potatoes and bananas. Cut out sugary foods and caffeine, and drink pure water only. Feed your brain a mixture of lecithin, wheat germ and brewer's yeast (take 2–3 tablespoons daily). You may sprinkle it on cereal or oatmeal.

Supplement support for depression

The following natural supplements have been used with great success:

- 5-HTP: Natural Prozac, naturally increases serotonin levels. It is important in the formation of neurotransmitters in the brain. (NOTE: 5-HTP should not be taken in conjunction with SSRI medication.)

- St. John's wort: A natural antidepressant; good for mild to moderate depression; take 300 mg three times daily. (NOTE: St. John's wort should not be taken in conjunction with SSRI medication.)

- SAM-e: 400 mg daily has been a blessing to depression sufferers, relieving both depression and pain in many instances.

- Liquid serotonin: One of the neurotransmitters in the brain that helps us to feel calm and relaxed. It can be used when the serotonin level in the brain is depleted from depression and is safe at any time of the day or night and by all ages. For optimal effectiveness, it should be used in conjunction with other amino acids.

- Brain Link Complex: A complete amino acid complex powder that creates neurotransmitter links for enhanced brain function. Brain Link was formulated by Billie J. Sahley. I feel that it is the most complete neurotransmitter formula available today.

- Coenzyme Q_{10}: Stimulates immunity and helps decrease immunodeficiency in times of chronic anxiety, depression and grief.

- Carlson ACES: Antioxidants are crucial when you are battling emotional illness.

- Tyrosine: Needed for brain function. This amino acid is excellent for people who have prolonged and intense stress. Uncontrollable stress may be prevented or reversed if tyrosine is taken either in capsule form or obtained in the diet. (NOTE: If you are taking an MAO inhibitor drug, you should not take tyrosine because it can raise your blood pressure. Take the thyroid test found in the self-test section of this book if you suspect your thyroid is sluggish. Follow the recommendations listed, and see your healthcare professional.)

Dermatitis

Dermatitis refers to an inflammation of the skin and can be caused by allergies, perfumes, poison ivy, cosmetics, genetic predisposition, metals or metal alloys as well as stress and chronic tension. Because *Staphylococcus aureus* infection is possible with any type of dermatitis, you may require antibiotics. See your doctor if your condition does not respond to dietary changes and supplement recommendations.

Definition

Dermatitis is an inflammation of the skin causing eczema, allergic or contact dermatitis, seborrhea, poison ivy, etc.

Symptoms

Symptoms include itching, redness, flaking, scaling and lesions that may blister, weep and ooze. Eczema is often associated with asthma.

Dietary considerations

Consider a detoxification program (Nature's Secret Ultimate Cleanse). Eat brown rice and millet. Focus on pineapples, celery, green leafy vegetables, grapes, melons, onions and papaya. Avoid sugar, fried foods and white flower. Eliminate dairy completely. (Children especially are allergic to cow's milk.)

Keep a food journal to help determine the cause of flare-ups.

Supplement support for dermatitis

- B complex with extra B_{12} and biotin: 50 mg
- Glucosamine: Take as directed
- Licorice root
- Vitamin A: 25,000 IU daily
- Beta carotene: 25,000 IU daily
- Essential fatty acids
- Evening primrose oil[45]
- Vitamin D
- PABA: 200 mcg three times daily
- Chamomile in topical cream (acts as an anti-inflammatory)
- Milk thistle liquid extract
- Passionflower, valerian, hops (Anxiety Control 24: a formula from the Pain and Stress Center)
- Sleep Link for a good night's sleep (see Product Section)

Lifestyle choices

- Oatmeal baths (such as Aveeno) relieve itching.
- Cornstarch or baking soda applied to the skin after bathing will help keep the skin dry.
- Make sure that your laundry detergent is free of dyes and perfumes.
- Always moisturize after bathing.

   ❦   Use Cetaphil Soap and Lotion.

   ❦   Make sure that your cosmetics are not contributing to your problem.

   ❦   Do a liver flush to help promote skin health.

DIABETES—JUVENILE AND ADULT

More than seventeen million people suffer from diabetes in this country according to the U.S. Department of Health and Human Services.[46] Diabetes occurs when all of the sugar and carbohydrates that a person consumes are not used properly. The pancreas produces too much insulin, creating high blood sugar. Diabetes can be very dangerous, leading to heart and kidney disease, stroke, blindness, hypertension and even death. Jonathan Wright, M.D. recommends that diabetics totally eliminate refined sugar and sugar products from their diet. My clients feel wonderful after eliminating sugar from their lives.

Definition
Diabetes is a disease based in the pancreas that results in abnormally high blood sugar levels.

Symptoms
Symptoms of diabetes include dry itching skin, extreme thirst, frequent and excessive urination, obesity, hypertension, kidney problems, blurred vision, high blood sugar, constant hunger and sugar cravings.

Bloodshot eyes can also be a sign of diabetes. If your eyes are frequently bloodshot (red), consult your doctor. Some other causes of reddened eyes may be allergies and eyelid infections.

Dietary considerations
A healthy diet of high-fiber foods and chromium-rich foods such as eggs, brewer's yeast, onions, garlic, shiitake mushrooms and wheat germ is especially helpful in controlling diabetes. Eat salmon at least once a week for omega-3s, and avoid all fatty and fried foods. Also, avoid cow's milk and alcohol.

Sugar and diabetes
Sugar consumption inhibits immune function, starting just thirty minutes after consumption and lasting for more than five hours. Sugar gives you a lift that eventually brings you down lower than where you started. As little as 100 grams of sugar in any form—honey, table sugar, fructose or glucose—can reduce the ability of your immune system's army to engulf and destroy invaders. Instead of consuming sugar for energy as so many Americans do daily, for a healthier life try to consume complex carbohydrates like whole-grain bread, rice or potatoes. These foods will boost your energy and will not suppress your immune system.

Sugar is also a food we reach for in times of stress or tension. This is especially detrimental to health because it makes your system acidic and strips the body of stabilizing B vitamins. As our lifestyles become more and more hectic, we consume more and more sugar.

Sugar has also been implicated in the leading cause of death in America: heart disease. People who consume a high-sugar diet can develop high levels of blood fats, triglycerides and cholesterol. I have found in my clients with high triglycerides that sugar was their daily treat.

Once these clients were educated on the dangerous risk of heart disease from having a sweet tooth, they cleaned up their diets faster than you can imagine. Also, fat does not make you fat. Sugar does. Yes, sugar is stressing your entire body daily, making you feel tired and irritable, and, most importantly, contributing to a future of chronic disease.

There are other, more healthy ways to add sweetness to your life. I use Stevia Extract instead of white table sugar. You may also use honey, date sugar, maple syrup and fructose in *moderation.*

Sugar and hypoglycemia

The inverse of high blood sugar, diabetes, is low blood sugar, or hypoglycemia. Both diseases are known to be caused in part by excessive sugar consumption. Hypoglycemia is extremely common these days. I believe the increase of hypoglycemia is due to the high-carbohydrate, high-sugar foods that we crave in our stressful lives along with the fact that we consume little or no fiber. This type of eating overloads the pancreas, which in turn overproduces insulin to lower the blood sugar, which translates into low blood sugar or hypoglycemia. If you are consuming too much sugar on a daily basis, you may be setting yourself up for hypoglycemia.

Symptoms of hypoglycemia include rapid pulse, weakness, crying spells, cold sweats, heart palpitations, irritability, anxiety, poor concentration, twitching, fatigue, exhaustion and nightmares. If these symptoms are familiar to you, you must eat more fiber foods and cut back on simple sugars. Eat protein foods at each meal. It is imperative that you have a protein snack in between meals to help keep your blood sugar levels stable all day long.

Supplement support for eliminating sugar

Eliminating sugar will not be easy because it is very addictive. Here are some suggestions to make the adjustment easier.

- Chromium picolinate
- Pantothenic acid
- Stevia Extract as an herbal sweetener
- B complex
- High fiber: brown rice, for example
- Adrenal gland supplement
- Vitamin C
- Calcium and magnesium
- Whey protein shake each morning

DIABETES QUIZ

Since low blood sugar can predispose you to developing diabetes later in life, take this quiz to see if your sugar consumption may be affecting your level of health now as well as later on.

Yes No

❏ ❏ Do you have a family history of diabetes?

❏ ❏ Do you crave sweets at certain times of the day?

❏ ❏ When you are under stress, do you crave sweets?

❏ ❏ Do you consume ice cream, chocolate, pies, cakes, candy, etc. more than twice a week?

❏ ❏ Do you feel weak and shaky if your meal is delayed?

❏ ❏ Do you feel tense, uptight and nervous at certain times during the day?

❏ ❏ Do you crave colas or other sweetened soft drinks?

❏ ❏ Do you pay attention to low-fat foods while ignoring the higher sugar content typically found in them?

If you answered *yes* to four or more of these questions, your excess sugar consumption may be sending you into low blood sugar or hypoglycemia. This condition may cause you to become diabetic later on from a pancreas that is simply too worn out to produce the necessary insulin crucial for controlling blood sugar levels.

Health Update   The Breast Is Best

According to recent medical studies by Hans-Michael Dosch, infants given cow's milk formula during their first three months of life face an increased risk of diabetes later in life. The theory for what causes this risk is that cow's milk contains a protein called bovine serum albumin, which must be eliminated. Because it is similar to the proteins found in insulin-producing cells in the pancreas, the immune system attacks these healthy cells as well.[47] Based upon Dr. Dosch's study, mothers should strive to breast-feed their babies for at least the first three months of life.

DIVERTICULOSIS

This common condition affects about 40 percent of Americans over the age of fifty.[48] A diet consisting of too many refined foods and a lack of fiber lead to a weakened colon wall, with a resultant formation of pouches. A low-fiber diet also leads to chronic constipation and gas, which worsens the condition. Emotional stress can cause colon spasms, and obesity causes a prolapsed colon structure. If the diet is not improved and emotional stress not addressed, diverticulosis may develop into diverticulitis, with symptoms that include abdominal cramping and pain, distention, diarrhea and rectal bleeding.

Definition

Diverticulosis is the development of multiple small pouches, called diverticula, in the wall of the large intestine. Diverticulitis, a more serious disease, occurs when the small pouches become infected and inflamed.

Symptoms

Symptoms include abdominal cramping, pain, distention, diarrhea and rectal bleeding.

Dietary considerations

- Add fiber to the diet to prevent constipation.
- Add yogurt.
- Eat lean protein (tofu, seafood, beans, brown rice).
- Eliminate dairy, fatty, fried or sugary foods.
- Do not eat nuts or seeds.
- Drink plenty of water, six to eight glasses per day.

Supplement support for diverticulosis

- B-complex vitamins
- Magnesium chloride liquid to reduce spasms
- Wild yam capsules
- Evening primrose oil
- L-glutamine
- Echinacea-goldenseal capsules
- L-theanine to reduce stress
- A daily green drink (Kyo-Green)
- Bio-K Liquid Acidophilus during acute phase, then Kyo-Dophilus capsules daily

Lifestyle choices

- Regular massage therapy
- Exercise, i.e., a good walking program
- A warm castor oil pack applied to abdomen three times weekly

EARACHES

This painful condition can be caused by several factors. An earache can be a residual effect of a bronchial infection, flu or cold that has settled in the ear. Other causes include food allergies (especially dairy) and too many mucus-producing foods. In adults, the most common cause of earache is swimmer's ear, which involves the outer ear canal. Children frequently suffer from middle ear infections and are placed on powerful antibiotics. This in turn may cause thrush or candidiasis. Breast-feeding your children helps to safeguard them against ear infections by boosting immunity and preventing allergies.

Definition
An earache is any pain or pressure in or around the ear.

Symptoms
Symptoms include acute, stabbing pain in the ear, eustachian tube or mastoid area; swelling; inflammation and slight fever. In children, temporary hearing loss, nausea, vomiting and a pus discharge from the ear may occur. Many children have tubes placed in the ear for drainage purposes. Ultimately, this treatment may damage hearing. Strengthening the immune system is your best defense.

Dietary considerations
Eliminate all dairy, fruit juice, fried foods, milk and sugars. Read all food labels, and avoid additives like MSG. Drink eight to ten glasses of water daily. Also have a green drink each day.

Supplement support for earaches
- For swimmer's ear: Mix 1 oz distilled white vinegar and 70 percent isopropyl alcohol in a dropper bottle. Place three drops into the ear canal and then let it drain out. Repeat two times daily.
- Grapefruit seed extract capsules
- Vitamin C
- Beta glucan
- Echinacea extract

Lifestyle choices
- Ear candling is effective for preventative maintenance. (Refer to directions on page 225.)
- Place a few drops of Kyolic Garlic liquid and warm olive oil in the ear canal or press onion juice out on a cotton ball and place it in ear canal.
- Massage area around ear including the neck. Pull on ear lobes ten times to stimulate circulation.

NOTE: See your physician if no improvement is noted, if hearing loss worsens or if fever persists.

Health Update   Listen Up! Earlobes
Speak Volumes

Creased earlobes are a better predicator of future heart trouble than diabetes, high blood pressure, smoking, high cholesterol, family history of coronary disease or obesity. In a study, having one creased earlobe raised the risk by 33 percent. Having both earlobes creased raised the risk by 77 percent. The link between earlobe creases and heart disease is not yet thoroughly understood. But if you have them, you need to take dietary and lifestyle measures to lower your risk.[49]

Eating Disorders—Anorexia/Bulimia

Today's society has placed much emphasis on being thin. For a young woman, the pressure to be thin can be overwhelming. The pages of magazines are filled with waif-like women who are often made even thinner by computer enhancement. Many American teenage girls are suffering from distorted body image. These disorders are extremely difficult to overcome and may even be fatal.

Anorexia is characterized by self-starvation. Bulimia is characterized by binge-purge cycles (eating extremely large quantities of food and, shortly after, vomiting to purge it from the body). Men are not excluded from either of these disorders. With the huge fitness craze that has taken place in the past twenty years, more men have taken up bodybuilding and weight training. The pressure to be fit and "buff" has led to the same distorted thinking in men that women suffer. It has been said that deep-seated emotional issues are at the root of these two disorders. Counseling is definitely recommended! The key to recovery is helping to raise the self-esteem of the sufferer. Low self-esteem is always implicated in the development of these disorders.

Definition
An eating disorder is any disorder that results in long-term, obsessive behavior relating to food or the body.

Symptoms
Symptoms include low blood pressure, irritable and aggressive behavior, constipation, cold hands and feet, dry skin, dull eyes, no menstrual period, eroded tooth enamel (from vomiting), low pulse rate, weakness and depression.

Amino Acids to Combat Addictions

Brain Neurotransmitter	Function	Drugs That Affect Neurotransmitter	Neurotransmitter Deficiencies Result	Amino Acid Supplement
Norepinephrine	Arousal, energy, drive	Cocaine, speed, caffeine, tobacco, marijuana, alcohol, sugar	Lack of drive, depression, lack of energy	L-tyrosine, L-phenylalanine
GABA (gamma-amino butyric acid)	Staying calm	Valium, alcohol, marijuana, tobacco	Free-floating, anxiety, fearfulness, insecurity, can't relax or sleep, unexplained panic	L-glutamine, GABA
Endorphins	Psychological and physical pain relief, pleasure, reward, good feelings toward others, loving feelings	Heroin, marijuana, alcohol, sugar, tobacco	Overly sensitive, feelings of incompleteness, anhedonia (inability to experience pleasure in a normal way), world looks colorless, inability to love	dL-phenylalanine
Serotonin	Emotional stability, pain tolerance, confidence	Sugar, marijuana, ecstasy, tobacco	Depression, obsession, worry, low self-esteem, sleep problems, sweet cravings, irritability	L-tryptophan

Dietary considerations

Eat foods that are powerhouses, such as high-protein vegetables, high-grain cereals, yogurt and carrot juice.

Add fresh fruits and vegetables (they are loaded with vitamins and minerals). Drink whey protein drinks and Kyo-Green daily. Eliminate sugars and all junk foods.

Supplement support for eating disorders

- Vital K–Potassium liquid
- 5-HTP for mood elevation
- B complex
- GABA
- Enzymedica's Digest
- Royal jelly
- Multimineral formula

Amino acids to help combat addictions

Alcoholics, anorexics and bulimics who are nutritionally depleted often have severe deficiencies of important brain neurotransmitters that govern mood and emotion. Amino acid supplementation is important to rebalancing patients' brain chemistries while recovering. (See chart on page 157.) Withdrawal from addictive substances should be supervised by a qualified health expert.

Eczema

Definition

Eczema is a group of skin conditions that cause dry, hot, itchy skin that occasionally bleeds and becomes raw.

Symptoms

Symptoms include severe itching and chronic, silvery-red skin rash found on the neck, knees, elbows and wrists.

FOR NATURAL REMEDIES SEE DERMATITIS

Endometriosis

This painful condition is on the rise. It is caused by dominant estrogen levels and deficient progesterone, yeast infections and prostaglandin imbalance, as well as excessive caffeine and alcohol, magnesium deficiency, hypoglycemia and sexually transmitted diseases (vaginal warts and chlamydia). Endometriosis increases the risk of uterine and breast fibroids, and many times may lead to hysterectomy. The keys for improvement are hormonal rebalancing, enhancing the immune response and addressing liver health. Endometriosis often calms down after menopause or after the hormones are rebalanced.

Definition

Endometriosis is a condition in which some of the inner lining of the uterus becomes implanted on other pelvic organs.

Symptoms

Symptoms include irritable bowel syndrome, cramping, abdominal and rectal pain, heavy periods, constipation or diarrhea.

Dietary considerations

Eat lots of fresh foods, especially fruits and vegetables. Include soy products, if you are not allergic to them, to balance estrogen. Avoiding sugar, caffeine, alcohol, animal fats, chocolate, fried foods and dairy foods will increase estrogen levels.

Supplement support for endometriosis

- Dr. Janet's Woman's Balance Formula (progesterone cream)
- Dandelion root extract
- Milk thistle extract
- B complex
- GABA
- Coenzyme Q$_{10}$
- Ester C: 3000 mg
- Kelp tablets for thyroid balance
- Flax oil

Lifestyle choices

- Warm castor oil packs on abdomen
- Regular massage therapy
- Regular exercise
- Early morning sunlight

EPSTEIN-BARR VIRUS

Definition

Epstein-Barr is a virus that causes mononucleosis.

Symptoms

Symptoms include fatigue, mental or physical exhaustion, and no energy or enthusiasm to do anything.

FOR NATURAL REMEDIES SEE CHRONIC FATIGUE SYNDROME

EYE HEALTH/PROBLEMS

It has been said that the eyes are the "windows to the soul." When you are not well or are suffering from unrest, the eyes are many times the first indication that something is wrong. Hence, the phrase, "I can see it in your eyes." Eye disorders range from mild discomfort (dry, itchy, tired, watery) to severe diseases, which include infection, cataracts, glaucoma, yellowing of the eyes (liver disease) and droopy eyes *(Myasthenia Gravis)*. Differences in pupil size can indicate tumor or concussion, bulging eyes can indicate thyroid problems, and red streaks in the eyes and blurring can indicate hypertension or even diabetes. In natural medicine, the belief is that a healthy liver plays a key role in eye health.

Definition
Eye health problems are defined as any degeneration of vision.

Symptoms
Symptoms included blurred vision, headaches, floaters, spots, redness and itching of eyes.

Dietary considerations
Drink plenty of water and eat plenty of carrots, yams, cantaloupes, onions, broccoli and other fruits and vegetables. Remember that colorful foods promote eyesight. Drink carrot juice and eat sunflower seeds. Be sure to reduce sugar intake.

Supplement support for eye health
- B complex
- Bilberry extract (improves day and night vision)
- Daily green drink (Kyo-Green)
- Eyebright
- Visual Eyes (Source Naturals)
- Multivitamin/mineral to insure you receive all of the essentials
- Carlson's ACES + Zinc for antioxidant protection
- Gingko biloba: circulation
- Chromium picolinate: sugar balance
- Dandelion tea: liver health
- Milk thistle extract: liver health
- Homeopathic Similasan natural eye drops for allergy or red eyes (800-426-1644).

Lifestyle choices
- Regular eye exams are recommended, especially for those over the age of thirty-five.
- Do a liver flush. (See page 223.)
- Place wet green tea bags over your eyes for blurred vision.

FIBROMYALGIA

Millions of Americans, mostly women, suffer from fibromyalgia. It is considered a stress-related immune disorder with the central cause being a low level of serotonin and reduced growth hormone. It is best described as an arthritic muscle disease.

Definition

Fibromyalgia is an arthritic muscle disease otherwise referred to as immune compromised musculo-skeletal pain.

Symptoms

Symptoms include painful, tender, recurrent aching points all over the body, diffuse musculo-skeletal pain and stiffness, fatigue, weakness, headaches, confusion, migraines, chronic bowel problems, poor sleep, nervous symptoms, hypoglycemia, shortness of breath, cardiovascular problems and allergies.

Causes

A compromised immune system often preceded by a stressful event, magnesium deficiency or possible viral connection, fibromyalgia is commonly associated with Mitral Valve Prolapse.

Dietary considerations

Follow an improved eating plan, avoiding sugars, fats, red meat and caffeine. Take Kyolic Garlic by Wakunaga daily.

Supplement support for fibromyalgia

For general symptoms, try royal jelly.

To reduce pain and inflammation try:

- Dr. Janet's Balanced by Nature Glucosamine Cream
- Quercetin, 1000 mg, and bromelain, 1500 mg

For brain balance try:

- Brain Link (amino acid powder)
- Gingko biloba
- GABA

For musculo-skeletal system try:

- L-carnitine, 1000 mg
- Magnesium capsules and Malic Acid
- B complex

Natural antidepressants to raise serotonin levels:

- SAM-e, 800 mg daily
- St. John's wort, 300 mg daily

For restful sleep try:

- Valerian root extract
- Kava
- Passionflower

To boost immunity try:

- Vitamin C, 3000 mg daily
- Coenzyme Q_{10}, 60 mg three times daily

Lifestyle choices

- ❦ Have a regular monthly massage.
- ❦ Listen to a relaxation tape.
- ❦ Take a stress-relieving bath. (See baths on pages 25 and 64.)
- ❦ Develop a meaningful prayer life.
- ❦ Read *Malic Acid and Magnesium for Fibromyalgia and Chronic Pain* by Billie J. Sahley, Ph.D., C.N.C.[50] (Call 800-669-2256 to order.)

Flu/Influenza

The flu can begin with symptoms that resemble the common cold, but the infection is generally more severe, highly contagious and longer lasting with lingering fatigue and weakness. Influenza can make a person more susceptible to pneumonia, sinus problems, bronchitis and ear infections.

People over the age of sixty can be seriously affected by the flu. It is the fifth leading cause of death in the elderly. Flu shots have not been as successful as hoped because viral strains constantly change and make one year's vaccine virtually obsolete.

Definition

Influenza (or flu) is an acute viral infection of the upper respiratory tract or digestive tract caused by a rhinovirus.

Symptoms

Symptoms include body aches, headache, fatigue and lethargy, fever, chills, hot flashes, dry or sore throat, cough, nausea and vomiting, diarrhea and abdominal pain. Weakness, loss of appetite and possibly a mildly depressed feeling can also accompany the illness.

Dietary considerations

Eat clear soups and grandma's chicken soup. Be sure to hydrate during the acute phase, consuming plenty of fluids such as spring water, herbal teas and fruit juices. Eliminate sugars and refined foods, and concentrate instead on fresh vegetables, steamed brown rice and whey protein shakes. Avoid pasteurized dairy foods as well as caffeine and alcohol. Also include power mushrooms—reishi, maitake and shiitake.

Supplement support for influenza

Acute phase:

- ❦ Ester C crystals to bowel tolerance (mix in water as directed)
- ❦ Grapefruit seed extract capsules
- ❦ Biotic silver
- ❦ Kyolic Garlic
- ❦ Echinacea extract
- ❦ Carlson ACES
- ❦ Zinc lozenges

Immune support:

- Astragalus
- NAC
- Coenzyme Q$_{10}$
- Kyo-Dophilus
- Thymus glandular
- Daily green drink

Lifestyle choices

At the first sign of flu, take echinacea and Oscillococcinum made by Boiron.

REST! Give your body a chance to heal! As you recover, gradually build your strength and have a massage once a week for one month. During the acute stage, take a sea salt and baking soda bath (see therapeutic baths on page 25) and sip room temperature water while bathing. To continue your progress, take a walk after dinner as your strength returns.

NOTE: Children's formulas are available at your local health food store. Look for alcohol-free echinacea and goldenseal liquid extracts, and put the drops in juice.

FOOD ALLERGIES

Food allergies are fast becoming as common as a cold or flu. This is because of all of the chemically altered, injected, sprayed and dyed foods that we ingest on a daily basis. Add to that stress, lack of sleep and enzyme deficiency from foods that are zapped by microwave preparation, and the allergies grow. Other causes include allergy to gluten-containing foods, inherited food sensitivities, MSG, sulfites and nitrates, food additives that are added to enhance color and flavor and cause a myriad of problems for sensitive individuals.

Definition

A food allergy is an autoimmune system body response to a certain food or an enzyme deficiency to digest a certain food.

Symptoms

Symptoms include irritability, headaches, candida, itchy, watery eyes, gas, constipation, sinus problems, bloated stomach, nausea, brain fog, heart palpitations, ringing in the ears, ear infections, weight gain, sweating, hives, IBS and arthritis symptoms.

Dietary considerations

For two weeks try the following sample diet. Make these foods a part of your daily menu. This is a fasting menu designed to prepare you for a rotation diet: brown rice; baked or broiled turkey, chicken or fish; herbal teas; steamed, broiled, raw or baked vegetables; vegetable and unsweetened, diluted fruit juices. Also add yogurt to your diet.

I suggest that you keep a food diary. After your two-week fasting menu, begin to add foods back and rotate your meals. Repeat foods only once every four days. For example, if you have a tomato stuffed with tuna on Monday, you should not have it again until Friday. This way you will be able to identify a food that you are sensitive to by evaluating symptoms. Continue to keep your food diary. As you rotate and eliminate, you will feel more energy, stabilized weight and a renewed feeling of well-being.

Avoid these common allergy foods:

- Peanuts
- Mushrooms
- Wheat
- Dairy
- Sugar
- Corn
- Eggs
- Soy
- Coffee
- Strawberries

Supplement support for food allergies

- Coenzyme Q$_{10}$: 100 mg daily
- Quercetin: 500 mg between meals
- Digest from Enzymedica
- Kyo-Dophilus from Wakunaga
- Ester C: 3,000 mg daily
- Adrenal glandular formula
- Milk thistle liquid extract
- Candex to eliminate candida yeast
- Liquid chlorophyll: 1 teaspoon in water before meals

Lifestyle choices

- Focus on stress management for better digestion, sleep and recuperative ability.

- If you have gained weight, even though you have not changed your eating habits, eliminate wheat from your diet for two weeks to see if your weight gain is allergy related.

- Keep a food diary, and record symptoms as you eliminate foods to determine the offenders.

- Use Coca's Pulse Test, developed by Arthur Coca, M.D., to identify allergens

- If symptoms do not improve, see an allergist and have skin prick or RAST tests done to determine what you are sensitive or allergic to.

Health Update — Coca's Pulse Test

Take your pulse when you wake up in the morning. Your pulse should be sixty to one hundred beats per minute. Take your pulse again after eating a suspected food that may be causing allergy symptoms. Wait fifteen to twenty minutes, and take your pulse again. If your pulse rate has increased by more than ten beats per minute, remove that food from your diet.

GALLBLADDER DISEASE/GALLSTONES

This problem is on the rise in America due in part to the poor diet Americans eat each day, filled with sugars and low in fiber, resulting in poor digestion. Over twenty million Americans have gallstones and/or gallbladder inflammation known as cholecystitis. The majority of sufferers are women; they account for 75 percent of the cases.[51]

The gallbladder helps digest fats by producing bile. If the gallbladder bile fluids become saturated with cholesterol, solid crystals form and eventually become gallstones. The key plan of attack is to increase bile solubility to reduce cholesterol levels. In addition, bile flow needs to be increased to aid the gallbladder in expelling small stones.

Definition

Gallbladder disease is an inflammation of the gallbladder caused by saturated bile known as gallstones.

Symptoms

Symptoms include pain in the upper right abdomen during an attack, nausea, cold sweats, possible fever, belching, anxiety, bloating, headache and anger. Some people report that the symptoms made them feel as if they were having a heart attack. The pain becomes more intense as the stones enlarge.

Causes

Causes include chronic indigestion from excessive refined sugar and dairy products, too many fried and fatty foods, food allergies, birth control pills and ERT, which cause an increase in cholesterol production, and sedentary lifestyle.

Dietary considerations

Eat smaller meals that are primarily vegetarian. Avoid red meat, dairy and eggs because they are high in saturated fats. Each morning take 1 tablespoon of honey and 2 tablespoons of apple cider vinegar in a glass of water. Drink six to eight glasses of water daily, and add lemon to each glass of water that you drink.

Supplement support for gallbladder disease

- Milk thistle liquid extract: for liver function
- Tumeric (curcumin): for inflammation
- B complex
- Chromium picolinate: 200 mcg daily (for weight over 150 pounds, 400 mcg daily)
- Choline and inositol: to regulate cholesterol levels
- Phosphatidylcholine: to regulate cholesterol levels
- Ester C: 3,000 mg daily
- Fiber supplement

> ❦   Taurine: keeps bile thinned
> ❦   Chamomile tea
> ❦   Acidophilus capsules (Kyo-Dophilus)

Lifestyle choices

> ❦   Do a liver flush (refer to page 223). CAUTION: This flush is *not* intended for people who have large stones. Consult your physician regarding advisability.
>
> ❦   Place a warm castor oil pack on the abdomen before bed.
>
> ❦   Start to exercise. Walking every night after dinner is wonderful for digestion and helps to reduce body fat.

Gastric Disease: Gastritis, Gastroenteritis and GERD

Gastritis, gastroenteritis and gastric ulcers are ulcerative disorders of the gastrointestinal tract. Ulcers are common in Americans because of our lifestyle. Stress, poor diets and long-term use of anti-inflammatory medications (NSAIDS) cause ulcers and gastrointestinal bleeding. A chronic sinus condition with postnasal drip also contributes to these diseases. The bacterium H. pylori has been implicated as well in the development of most ulcers.

With all of the stress, poor dietary habits, improper food combining and enzyme-deficient foods to which we are exposed, it is no wonder that gastric disease has risen sharply in the past two decades. GERD and hiatal hernias are extremely common.

Natural medicine has been very successful in alleviating all gastric diseases by supporting intestinal mucosa, enzyme activity and probiotic balance.

Definition

Gastric disease is characterized by inflammation of the stomach and intestinal tract; it also involves the leaking of stomach acid back into the lower esophagus and acid coming up into the throat.

Symptoms

Symptoms include excess gas, belching, bloating and heartburn. After eating, hiccups, regurgitation, pressure behind the breastbone, nervousness, diarrhea, high blood pressure and difficulty swallowing may be experienced. Sufferers also experience irritable bowel syndrome, sharp abdominal pains and chest pains, poor digestion and shortness of breath.

Gastric or peptic ulcers form open sores in the stomach or duodenum walls and cause burning, diarrhea, nausea, dark feces and bright red vomit (signs of duodenal ulcer).

Dietary considerations for all gastric diseases

Eat only small meals and chew all food well. Do not eat late at night.

During flare-ups, eat raw and lightly steamed vegetables. Avoid fried and spicy foods. If you have a hiatal hernia, you need to avoid chocolate, alcohol, red meat, coffee and carbonated beverages. Add therapeutic juices, such as freshly made carrot juice, carrot-cabbage juice and carrot-papaya juice, to your diet to heal the affected tissues.

Supplement support for gastric conditions

- Chamomile tea
- Pau d'arco tea
- MSM
- Gastro from Enzymedica
- Magnesium
- Purify from Enzymedica
- Glutamine powder: 500 mg three times daily
- Ester C: 3000 mg daily
- Kyo-Dophilus before meals
- Daily green drink

Lifestyle choices

- Do not eat when emotionally upset.
- Practice deep-breathing exercises to promote relaxation.
- Consider chiropractic treatment or massage therapy weekly until improvement is noticed.
- Do not lie down immediately after eating.
- Do not smoke.
- If you are overweight, plan to lose weight.
- Antacids can cause more problems in the long term. They may cause kidney stones and contribute to high blood pressure. Antacids that contain aluminum may also raise the risk of aluminum toxicity.
- Avoid NSAID medications, especially if you have an ulcer.

GOUT

Gout is an extremely painful form of arthritis. Many sufferers are middle-aged males who are obese. It is caused by the accumulation of too much uric acid in the blood, tissues and urine. While gout primarily affects the foot and big toe, the kidneys, fingers, joints and tendons can also be affected. A successful natural therapy protocol involves dietary changes and detoxification with focus on the kidneys to normalize uric acid levels in the tissues and blood. Gout is also linked to hypoglycemia and hypothyroidism.

Definition

Gout is arthritis of the toe and peripheral joints.

Symptoms

Symptoms include chills, fever, redness and swelling of the joint(s).

Dietary considerations

Eat fresh cherries, celery, broccoli, bananas and strawberries. Drink six to eight glasses of water daily and four to five glasses of black cherry juice. Avoid alcohol, caffeine, fried foods, sardines, anchovies, red meat, spinach, clams, oysters, lobster, mushrooms and liver.

Supplement support for gout

- Cherry juice extract capsules
- Vitamin C (Ascorbate C)
- Enzymedica's Purify
- Devil's claw
- Flax oil
- Chromium picolinate: 200 mcg daily
- Glycine: 500 mg daily
- B complex
- Quercetin
- Kyo-Green

Lifestyle choices

- Soak foot in apple cider vinegar for relief (thirty minutes) or take a bath with one quart of apple cider vinegar.
- Buy a juicer and begin to juice each day.
- Lose weight, and exercise to stimulate circulation.

Headaches: Migraines, Cluster

Headaches are common in these days of increased stress and tension. Headaches seem to occur most frequently in A-type personalities—people who are highly goal-oriented, perfectionists who demand a great deal from themselves and from those around them.

There are two basic types of headaches: those that are the result of stress and tension, and those that are brought on by a real physical cause. Stress control is the way to go when it comes to breaking the headache cycle. Physical causes include oral contraceptives and HRT, food allergies, sluggish liver, encephalitis, poor circulation, poor posture, TMJ, histamine reactions too much caffeine and magnesium deficiency.

Definition

Headaches are any mild to severe pain located in the head, characterized by throbbing or aching.

Symptoms

Common symptoms include head pain, aching in the temples and forehead accompanied by irritability and tension. Migraine and cluster headaches (vascular headaches) are the most painful and can involve the entire body. Migraine headaches often include nausea, vomiting, chills, diarrhea and sensitivity to light and smells. Cluster headaches are extremely painful and are centered over the forehead or eyes. They generally come on suddenly.

Dietary considerations

Eat turkey to boost serotonin levels, and add almonds, dark leafy greens, broccoli, pineapple and cherries. Avoid headache triggers such as alcohol, wine, beer, dairy foods, caffeine, sugar, chocolate, wheat, sulfites, nitrates, MSG and pizza. A cup of black coffee can relieve headache once it has begun.

Supplement support for headaches

- Nature's Secret Ultimate Cleanse to detoxify
- Green tea sweetened with Stevia
- Feverfew and gingko biloba
- Magnesium
- GABA and B complex to calm and relax
- Evening primrose oil
- Dr. Janet's Woman's Balance Formula (progesterone cream) for hormonal headaches
- Carlson's ACES
- Bromelain
- 5-HTP to calm stress
- DLPA for pain
- A daily green drink (Kyo-Green)

Lifestyle choices

- Massage therapy
- Aromatherapy using lavender oil
- Therapeutic baths with sea salt, baking soda and lavender oil
- Chiropractic treatment
- Deep breathing
- Exercise
- Ice pack applied to the back of the neck; for nausea, place ice pack on the throat.
- For tension headache, take a brisk walk and breathe deeply.
- Take time out to focus on relaxation every day.
- Laughter is the best medicine!
- Homeopathy: belladonna; bryonia; nux vomica

HEARING LOSS

One in ten Americans suffer from some form of hearing loss. Hearing loss is the third most common problem for people over the age of sixty-five. About 85 percent of hearing loss is related to ringing in the ears or tinnitus. Other causes of hearing loss include allergies, sinus inflammation, chronic bronchial mastoid inflammation, arteriosclerosis, excess ear wax, poor circulation, high blood pressure, metabolic imbalance, low immunity, autoimmune disease, hypoglycemia and a diet that consists of too many mucus-forming foods.[52]

Definition

Hearing loss is defined as the loss of ability to perceive sounds as compared with what would be considered normal due to tinnitus, ear malfunction and excess wax.

Symptoms

Symptoms include ringing in the ears and diminished ability to hear.

Dietary considerations

Eat as close to the "original garden" as possible, that is, whole grains, fresh fruit, vegetables and vegetable proteins. Drink six to eight glasses of water daily with fresh lemon for added benefit. Eliminate or limit intake of chocolate, caffeine and alcohol. And reduce or avoid sugars, salt and dairy foods.

Supplement support for hearing loss

- Beta carotene: 150,000 IU daily
- Ester C: 3,000 mg daily
- PCOs from grapeseed or pinebark: 100 mg three times daily
- Coenzyme Q_{10}: 30 mg daily
- Ginkgo biloba: 60 mg three times daily
- Nature's Secret Ultimate Oil
- Echinacea extract drops to fight infection
- Goldenseal: Use only one week at a time to fight infection
- Vitamin B_{12}: 2,500 mcg with folic acid
- Cayenne-ginger capsules for improved circulation
- Magnesium: 800 mg
- Glutamine: 1000 mg
- Multivitamin/mineral formula
- A daily green drink

Especially for ringing in the ears

- Mullein
- Hyssop
- Eucalyptus
- Ephedra
- Black cohosh
- Licorice extract
- Limit aspirin use

Lifestyle choices

- Ear candling (Refer to instructions on page 225.) NOTE: DO NOT EAR CANDLE BY YOURSELF!

- For earwax buildup, make a solution of vinegar, warm water and three drops of hydrogen peroxide. Drop into ear with a dropper. Wait one minute, then drain. Do this daily until you get relief.

🌿 For ear infection, place two to four drops of warm liquid Kyolic Garlic into the ear canal. Eliminate wheat and dairy because they are common food allergy triggers. You should notice a difference in two weeks.

🌿 If hearing loss becomes worse or does not improve, a professional evaluation is recommended.

HEART ATTACK AND RELATED HEART CONDITIONS

Definition

Heart attacks and heart conditions occur when the supply of blood to the heart is sharply reduced.

Symptoms

Symptoms include shortness of breath, nausea, vomiting, chest pressure, sweating, panic, high or low blood pressure and fatigue.

Risk factors for heart disease

Heart disease is the number one killer of Americans, claiming over the lives of 720,000 people each year.[53] See the chart below for risk factors associated with increased heart disease risk.

Some of the risk factors are beyond your control. However, the most dangerous risk factors are the ones that you can do something about: smoking, high blood pressure and high cholesterol. If you decide to take a "statin" drug to lower your cholesterol, keep in mind that these drugs also lower the levels of coenzyme Q_{10} in your body and, in addition, may cause liver damage.

I recommend that you supplement with coenzyme Q_{10} for cholesterol problems whether or not you are taking medication. Coenzyme Q_{10} actually helps prevent heart attacks, boosts immunity, lowers blood pressure, is a powerful antioxidant and relieves periodontal disease according to some studies.[54]

RISK FACTORS FOR HEART DISEASE

Males or postmenopausal women
Age
History of heart disease in the family
High cholesterol
Smoking
Obesity
Lack of exercise
Stress
High blood pressure

Dietary considerations

Diet can be your single most effective preventative measure against heart disease. Add garlic, onions, green tea, seafood, wheat germ, brewer's yeast, molasses and lecithin granules to your diet. Red wine with dinner (one or two glasses) can raise HDL levels and reduce stress.

Avoid red meat, soft drinks and fried, fatty, salty and sugary refined foods. Drink eight glasses of spring water daily. Also limit hydrogenated oils.

Supplement support for heart disease

The following recommendations have been successful in keeping cardio-vascular systems healthy.

- Taurine: 1,000 mg twice daily. Taurine helps to balance the calcium and potassium in the heart as well as increasing the function of the left ventricle without changing the blood pressure.

- Carnitine: 1,000 to 3,000 mg per day in divided doses for high cholesterol and high triglycerides. Many people ask me how to raise the HDL or "good cholesterol" levels. I have found that carnitine in the right doses can help to accomplish a desirable HDL level.

- Chromium picolinate: 200 mcg daily (400 mcg if you weigh over 150 pounds). Chromium helps to lower triglycerides and cholesterol while raising HDL levels.

- Magnesium: Most people with coronary artery disease or CAD are deficient in magnesium. Magnesium is crucial to a healthy heart. It acts as a muscle relaxant.

- Vitamin E: A very important antioxidant. When vitamin E is taken daily, studies have shown a lower risk of fatal heart attacks.

- Coenzyme Q_{10}: The recommended dose is 100 mg per day if you have CAD or high blood pressure. If you suffer from congestive heart failure, the dose is 300 to 500 mg per day.

- Anxiety Control: Take this product as directed on the bottle for anxiety or stress.

- Ester C: 2,000 to 5,000 mg per day in divided doses

- Hawthorn Berry: Take as directed on product label. Hawthorn helps to improve circulation of the blood to the heart by dilating blood vessels and relieving arterial spasms.

- Kyo-Green: Have a green drink daily for healthy blood chemistry.

- Garlic or aspirin therapy: Taken each day. Garlic is an alternative to aspirin and is at least as potent. Both thin the blood, thereby discouraging clots that can block arteries.

Heartburn

If you live with chronic heartburn and indigestion, chances are you are aging faster than normal because your body's energy is reduced, toxins have accumulated, allergic reactions have occurred, and your immune defenses are low. What's more, as we get older our digestion weakens because we produce less stomach acid. Without enough stomach acid (HCl) we cannot digest proteins well. Following some simple natural medicine remedies will definitely improve this condition. As your digestion normalizes, you will notice that almost everything will improve. You will have more energy, sleep better and feel lighter and more energetic.

Definition
Heartburn is a burning sensation in the chest that occurs when hydrochloric acid from the stomach backs up into the esophagus.

Symptoms
Symptoms include a burning sensation in the stomach and/or the chest.

Causes
Causes of heartburn include stress, excessive consumption of spicy, fatty and fried foods, alcohol, coffee, citrus fruits, chocolate, hiatal hernia, ulcers, gallbladder problems, allergies and enzyme deficiency. Yeast overgrowth from antibiotic therapy, overeating and poor food combining also contribute.

Dietary considerations
Avoid onions, chocolate, citrus fruits, coffee, alcohol, spicy foods, tomato sauce, milk and soft drinks. Pineapple aids digestion.

FOOD COMBINING GUIDELINES

Digestion is optimal when foods are eaten together that have the same approximate digestion time. To facilitate optimal digestion, follow these guidelines:

- Proteins are eaten alone.
- Vegetables are eaten with grains and legumes.
- Starches and proteins should not be eaten together (rice can be eaten with protein.)
- Digestive enzymes at a meal will enhance digestion in addition to the above recommendations.

Supplement support for heartburn

- ❦ Ginger absorbs excess stomach acid.
- ❦ Slippery elm soothes the mucous membranes of the gastrointestinal tract.
- ❦ Fennel controls gas and bloating.
- ❦ Take vitamin B_{12} for digestion and assimilation.
- ❦ Acidophilus replaces healthy bowel flora.
- ❦ Water and apple cider vinegar: 1 teaspoon apple cider vinegar to one-half glass of water counteracts heartburn.
- ❦ Enzymatic therapy DGL tablets: Take to soothe the burn until your system rebalances.
- ❦ Have a green drink (such as Kyo-Green) daily.
- ❦ Take a probiotic supplement each day such as Bio-K or Kyo-Dophilus.

Lifestyle choices

Try not to eat when you are stressed or upset as this only makes digestion harder. Have a cup of peppermint or mint medley tea from Celestial Seasons to help complete digestion before you go to bed.

Health Update   Help for Heartburn

Lying on your left side keeps the stomach below the esophagus, which can help prevent and relieve heartburn by helping to keep the esophagus acid-free. At the first sign of heartburn, drink an 8-ounce glass of water.

HOW TO CHOOSE ENZYMES

It is important to understand that there are two sources for supplemental enzymes: plants and animals. Enzymes taken from the pancreas of an animal (pancreatic enzymes) may have been taken from an animal with poor health, posing obvious risks. In addition, they are not as digestively active as plant enzymes. Enzymes from a plant source are superior because plant enzymes become active as soon as they enter the body. In addition, they work throughout the entire digestive system and in the blood.

Look for appropriate codes approved by the FDA to insure active enzyme activity, and avoid products with fillers and cellulose added to the formula. The system for determining enzyme potency used by the American Food Industry is derived from the Food and Chemical Code or FCC. You should find an enzyme supplier that measures and reports the enzyme product levels in FCC units.

I recommend Enzymedica, a wonderful company located in Punta Gorda, Florida, that manufactures a superior line of enzymes. I use them exclusively. They meet all of the criteria for activity and potency. Furthermore, they have formulas specifically tailored to the four deficiency syndromes.

HOW TO TAKE ENZYMES

In order for the plant enzymes to provide maximum benefits during the digestion process, they need to be taken when their activity will be compatible with what is occurring during digestion. I instruct my clients to take their enzymes at the beginning of the meal; the rate of efficiency will not be as good at the end of a meal when acidity has already built up during the digestive process. According to "The White Paper" by Dr. M. Mamadou, microbiologist and enzymologist, it is recommended that oral enzymes be taken at the beginning of the meal, halfway during the meal and at the end of the meal for complete assimilation.

HEMORRHOIDS

This condition may not find its way into your daily conversation, but it certainly gets a lot of attention these days because of the increase in people who suffer from it. Again, it is caused by poor diets filled with low fiber and refined foods. In addition, sitting all day in front of computer screens, not drinking enough water, pregnancy, system toxicity, painkillers, obesity and allergies contribute to this painful condition.

Most of the time constipation plays a large part in the development of hemorrhoids as well. This being the case, I recommend you follow the guidelines listed for constipation in addition to the recommendations listed here. Natural medicine has been successful in alleviating hemorrhoids by diet changes, adequate hydration and daily exercise.

Definition
Hemorrhoids are clusters of swollen veins in the lining of the anus, usually accompanied by constipation.

Symptoms
Symptoms include itching and rectal bleeding associated with bowel movements, inflammation and constipation.

Dietary considerations
Eat fiber foods daily, such as bran, vegetables, dried fruit and cherries. Eat small meals to take stress off of the bowel. Take 1 tablespoon of olive or flaxseed oil before each meal. And drink eight to ten glasses of water daily. Avoid caffeine, sugar and low-fiber, refined foods.

Supplement support for hemorrhoids

- ❦ Enzymatic therapy: Hemotome
- ❦ Vitamin E: 400 IU
- ❦ Ester C: 3000 mg daily
- ❦ Bioforce Hemorrhoid Relief
- ❦ Milk thistle extract
- ❦ Colon Cleanz to alleviate constipation as needed
- ❦ Bromelain
- ❦ Vitamin K if bleeding is present
- ❦ Magnesium gel caps: 400 mg at bedtime as a stool softener and muscle relaxant
- ❦ Carlson's ACES
- ❦ A daily green drink

Lifestyle choices

- ❦ Take a brisk thirty-minute walk daily to promote healthy circulation.
- ❦ If you are overweight, try to lose weight.
- ❦ Take a warm sitz bath.
- ❦ Use ice packs and witch hazel to help to cool the pain and inflammation until improvement comes from natural remedies.
- ❦ Take the bowel function test on page 224. Add fiber as needed with plenty of water until you score an "A" on the test. This will give your condition a chance to heal.

HEPATITIS

Natural medicine's goal is to regenerate the liver and arrest the hepatitis virus while at the same time strengthen the body. Persons most at risk for hepatitis in all forms are medical workers, blood transfusion recipients (screening techniques have improved dramatically), dentists and dental workers and intravenous drug users.

Definition

Hepatitis is defined as an inflammation of the liver caused by one of five hepatitis viruses and by parasites and toxic reactions to drugs, alcohol and chemicals.

Symptoms

Symptoms of hepatitis include great fatigue and lethargy coupled with flu-like symptoms; enlarged, congested, tender and sluggish liver; nausea; gray stools; vomiting; skin jaundice; histamine itching; fever; loss of appetite; dark urine and elevated liver enzymes

Dietary considerations

For two or three weeks consume raw fruits and vegetables. Avoid fats, sugars and highly processed foods. In addition, avoid animal protein, raw fish and shellfish. Add artichokes to your diet; they protect the liver. Drink six to eight glasses of water daily, adding fresh lemon for extra liver cleansing benefit.

FIVE CATEGORIES OF HEPATITIS	
Hepatitis A	Otherwise known as infectious hepatitis, usually spread through person-to-person contact, often spread through blood or feces. Once you have contracted hepatitis A and recovered from it, you develop immunity to it.
Hepatitis B	Sexually transmitted as well as carried through transfused blood, saliva and dirty needles. Most cases of hepatitis B go undetected or are unrecognized. It can become chronic and can scar the liver, leading to cirrhosis of the liver or cancer, which can be fatal.
Hepatitis C	Usually develops after a blood transfusion with tainted or infected blood. However, it can also be contracted through sexual contact and IV drug use.
Hepatitis D	Associated with the cytomegalovirus and the Epstein-Barr virus.
Other	Less common forms include Non-A, Non-B and hepatitis E. All three are highly contagious.

Supplement support for hepatitis

For liver support and immune enhancement:

- Milk thistle extract
- B complex
- Licorice root: antiviral
- Coenzyme Q_{10}: 100 mg daily
- Dandelion root extract
- Astragalus
- Kyo-Dophilus or Bio-K (acidophilus)

To discourage viral replication:

- Grapefruit seed extract
- Echinacea
- St. John's wort
- Burdock: cleanses the liver

To heal the liver:

- L-carnitine
- Purify from Enzymedica
- Vitamin E
- Carlson's ACES

- ꙮ   Calcium: 1,500 mg daily, very important for blood clotting
- ꙮ   Magnesium: 1,000 mg daily, very important for blood clotting
- ꙮ   Primrose oil: essential fatty acid
- ꙮ   Daily green drink (Kyo-Green)
- ꙮ   Power mushrooms—maitake, shiitake and reishi—to boost immunity

Lifestyle choices

The good news about hepatitis is that natural medicine has had wonderful success in stopping viral replication and in regenerating the liver. Here are some lifestyle choices you can make that will help:

- ꙮ   Place warm castor oil packs on liver area.
- ꙮ   Make sure to rest enough.
- ꙮ   Do not drink alcohol.
- ꙮ   If you are the caregiver for a hepatitis patient, be sure to wash your hands and clothing often, and wash bed linens separately with bleach.

Health Update — Hepatitis B: Who Should Be Vaccinated?

International travelers
Doctors, nurses, paramedics
Firefighters, policemen
Morticians, embalmers
Patients and staff members at institutions for the mentally handi-
    capped
Ethnic groups with high rates of hepatitis B infections (Chinese, Native
    American, African American, Hispanic, American Eskimo)
Intravenous drug users
Persons living with or having sex with a hepatitis B carrier[55]

Health Update — Hepatitis A Vaccine

If you are a traveler under the age of fifty, you should consider getting the Havrix or Vaqta vaccine if you expect to take more than two extended trips to Eastern Europe, tropical developing countries or Persia within the next ten years. If you are going only once and plan to stay ten days or less, gamma globulin shots are a less expensive alternative. Talk to your doctor if you want to explore it further or if you are over fifty.[56]

Hiatal Hernia

This is a bothersome condition that is caused by an opening in the diaphragm that allows a protrusion of the upper part of the stomach into the esophagus. The uncomfortable symptoms include acid reflux, burning and inflammation. Please refer to the section on gastric diseases for more information.

Definition
   A hiatal hernia is a painful condition in which part of the stomach protrudes through the diaphragm wall.

Symptoms
   Symptoms include a feeling of fullness, acid reflux, anxiety and bloating.

Dietary considerations
   Eat several small meals daily, and never lie down right after a meal. Avoid the following foods that aggravate the condition: coffee, cola, tea, chocolate, lemons, tomato juice, grapefruit, oranges and spicy foods. Do not drink with your meals. Waiting to drink liquids after eating will help you digest your food better. Do not put ice in your beverages, as that will also adversely affect digestion.

Supplement support for hiatal hernia

   ❦ Plant enzymes with each meal
   ❦ Kyo-Green or liquid chlorophyll
   ❦ Kyo-Dophilus or an acidophilus supplement
   ❦ Chamomile tea at bedtime

SEE GASTRIC DISEASES

High Blood Pressure (Hypertension)

This condition is often called the *silent killer* because a person can be suffering from high blood pressure and not have any noticeable symptoms. The exact cause is sometimes hard to pinpoint as well. Contributing factors are heredity, high cholesterol, smoking, stress, high sodium intake, alcohol intake and obesity.
   Secondary hypertension can be caused by pregnancy, birth control pills, diabetes, kidney disease, arteriosclerosis, congestive heart failure and exposure to heavy metals. The incidence of high blood pressure increases with age, so frequent monitoring is suggested. Left untreated, life span is reduced.

Definition
   High blood pressure is blood pressure over 140 mm/hg systolic and over 90 mm/hg diastolic.

Symptoms
   Symptoms include dizziness, headache, irritability, bloodshot eyes and edema.

Dietary considerations

Eat a high-fiber diet, and add garlic, celery, olive oil and flaxseed oil to the diet. Avoid caffeine—it raises blood pressure. Reduce salt as it promotes fluid retention, which increases blood pressure. Avoid soy sauce, MSG and canned vegetables. Avoid smoked and aged cheeses and meats, chocolate, canned broths and animal fats. Limit sugar intake—it can increase sodium retention.

Supplement support for high blood pressure

- Arjuna bark: 500 mg three times daily
- Magnesium: 400–800 mg daily
- Hawthorn: 100–250 mg three times daily
- Vitamin E: 100 IU daily, may be increased to 400–800 IU daily
- B-complex vitamins
- Calcium (Citrate): 1000 mg daily
- Potassium (as directed on product label)
- Fiber supplement
- Milk thistle for liver function
- Garlic: inhibits platelet aggregation
- Valerian root: for stress
- Black cohosh: calms the cardiovascular system
- Cayenne: blood pressure normalizer

HEALTH FLASH: FORGIVENESS LOWERS BLOOD PRESSURE

According to a study at Florida Hospital in Orlando, Florida, conducted by head researcher Dick Tibetts, a group of hypertension patients took an eight-week forgiveness-training program. The patients who took forgiveness training had lower blood pressure than the control group who did not. The most dramatic reductions in blood pressure occurred in people who began the program with many anger issues.

Lifestyle choices

- Keep stress to a minimum.
- Have regular massage therapy.
- Prayerful meditation daily helps to diffuse stress.
- Use lavender aromatherapy.
- Practice deep breathing.
- Exercise to reduce stress and lose weight (check with your doctor for clearance); walking is ideal. Also, avoid heavy lifting.
- Drinking hard water lowers blood pressure; soft water is high in sodium and raises it. Soft water is associated with heart disease. Drink bottled water if you have a water softener at home.

    ❦   Purchase a blood pressure monitor and keep a daily journal of blood pressure readings. This will help you determine your rate of progress.

    ❦   Do not drink alcohol. It causes an immediate rise in blood pressure and adrenaline.

STAGES OF HYPERTENSION

Hypertension is ranked in the following stages:

	Systolic	*Diastolic*
Normal	120	80
Stage I	140 to 159	90 to 99
Stage II	160 to 179	100 to 109
Stage III	180 to 209	110 to 119
Stage IV	210 or higher	120 or higher

Even Stage I hypertension can cause serious health problems, increasing your chances of stroke, heart attack, kidney failure and more. Take immediate steps to lower your blood pressure if your reading is higher than 120/80.

HORMONAL IMBALANCE

Definition
In men, hormonal imbalance is defined as andropause, impotence or prostate health: In women, hormonal imbalance is estrogen dominance or post-hysterectomy/menopause.
SEE MENOPAUSE, PMS AND ANDROPAUSE

HYPOGLYCEMIA/LOW BLOOD SUGAR

There seems to be an epidemic of low blood sugar (hypoglycemia) in America these days because of our poor diets filled with sugar, alcohol, soft drinks, simple carbohydrates, caffeine, chocolate and coffee. Hypoglycemia may take a while to diagnose because the symptoms resemble those of other diseases, such as allergies, chronic fatigue syndrome, asthma, neurological problems, weight problems, thyroid and pituitary disorders, kidney disease and adrenal exhaustion. A Glucose Tolerance Test can be performed to help determine whether or not low blood sugar is causing your symptoms. Often dietary changes alone can resolve this condition.

Definition

Hypoglycemia is a condition in which the pancreas overreacts to repeated high sugar intake by producing too much insulin. This in turn causes the blood sugar to lower too much.

Symptoms

Symptoms include dizziness, headache, irritability, fainting spells, anxiety, depression, insomnia, craving for sweets, confusion, weakness in the legs and more. These symptoms may occur for a few hours after eating sweets or fats.

Dietary considerations

Eat a high-fiber diet, with some form of protein at each meal. Eat beans, brown rice, vegetables, low-fat cottage cheese, tofu, yogurt, nuts, seeds, avocados, almond butter and soy or rice cheese.

Avoid sweet fruit juices. Dilute them 50/50 with water. Eliminate sugar, soft drinks, alcohol and refined and processed foods.

Supplement support for hypoglycemia

- Multivitamin/mineral formula
- Have a green drink (Kyo-Green) midmorning
- Chromium picolinate: 200 mcg (400 mcg if you are over 150 pounds)
- Vitamin B complex
- Extra pantothenic acid
- Magnesium: 400–800 mg daily in divided doses
- Vitamin C: 3,000 mg daily
- Stevia liquid extract as an herbal sweetener
- L-glutamine: 1000 mg daily to reduce sugar cravings
- L-carnitine: energizes the body
- Milk thistle and dandelion root for liver health
- Adrenal glandular formula
- A protein shake each day to help keep blood sugar stabilized

Lifestyle choices

- Reduce stress
- Exercise
- Massage therapy

HYPOTHYROIDISM

This condition currently affects over five million Americans. Women make up the largest percentage of sufferers, usually between the ages of thirty and fifty.[57]

Definition

Hypothyroidism is the deficiency of the thyroid gland in its production of thyroid hormone.

Symptoms

Symptoms of this often-diagnosed disease include profound fatigue, weight gain with slow metabolism, depression, cold hands and feet, constipation, hair thinning or loss and enlarged thyroid gland. If you can relate to any of these symptoms, have a simple blood test performed to check your TSH, T3 and T4 levels.

SELF-TEST FOR UNDERACTIVE THYROID

To test yourself for an underactive thyroid, take this self test developed by Broda Barnes. Keep a basal thermometer by your bedside. Before retiring, shake down the thermometer and place it within easy reach of your bed. In the morning, before arising, lie still and place the thermometer under your armpit for ten minutes. Be sure to lie very still! Any motion can upset the reading. Repeat this procedure for seven to ten days consecutively.

Females should not take a reading during the first few days of their menstrual cycle or at the middle day of their monthly cycle because body temperature fluctuates during those times. A normal reading is between 97.8 and 98.2. A temperature below 97.6 degrees Fahrenheit may indicate low thyroid function. Record your readings for the next ten days.

Date	Temperature
____	_____
____	_____
____	_____
____	_____
____	_____
____	_____
____	_____
____	_____
____	_____

Dietary considerations

Avoid foods that suppress thyroid function, such as peanuts, mustard, millet, soy and cabbage. These foods prevent iodine use in the body. Iodine-rich foods, such as mushrooms, garlic and onions, are excellent for thyroid function. Make sure you use salt or herb salt that contains iodine.

Supplement support for hypothyroidism

If you are not currently on thyroid medication, or if your condition is mild, you may use the following natural supplements to increase thyroid function:

   ❦   Kelp tablets as a natural source of iodine (as directed on the bottle)

- ❧ Core Level Thyroid from Nutri-West of Florida
- ❧ Antioxidants to protect the thyroid gland
- ❧ Coenzyme Q_{10}: 100 mg daily
- ❧ Carlson ACES
- ❧ Wakunaga's Neurologic: for memory improvement
- ❧ To enhance thyroid function especially during perimenopause and menopause, use Dr. Janet's Balanced by Nature Progesterone Cream as directed.

Take the appropriate supplement recommendations, and take a thirty-minute walk to stimulate your metabolism. See your healthcare provider if you suspect a sluggish thyroid. Problems with the thyroid can be the cause of many chronic and recurring illnesses and fatigue.

Your thyroid gland is the thermostat of your body. It produces hormones to help keep your metabolic rate stable and to keep energy-producing and energy-using processes in balance. If it is depleted or deficient, the rest of the body functions improperly, which leads to lower immunity. Thyroid problems can cause many recurring illnesses and fatigue.

If your temperature is consistently below 97.6, you should add the following supplements to your health-building program:

- ❧ Kelp: contains iodine
- ❧ Raw thyroid glandular: helps to replace deficient thyroid hormone
- ❧ B-complex vitamin: helps improve thyroid function and immune function
- ❧ Essential fatty acids: necessary for proper thyroid gland function
- ❧ See your physician for Armor Thyroid, available by prescription only.

IMMUNE SYSTEM HEALTH

In today's society, it is becoming increasingly difficult to keep our immune system strong. Without a strong immune system, we are more susceptible to illness. Our immune systems fight against many pathogens on a daily basis, such as yeast, parasites, fungi and viruses. They also combat many antigens such as pollen, chemicals, drugs, malignant cells and more.

The immune system is the greatest pharmacy in the world, making more than one hundred billion types of medicines known as antibodies to attack just about any unwanted germ or virus that enters our body. Best of all, all of the medicines made by our *internal pharmacy* do not produce side effects. In addition to being the most powerful healing agents known to man, they are free—or almost.

Your immune system has only one requirement: receiving the right raw materials to produce the internal medicines to safeguard you from illness. The following recommendations will help you to fortify yourself in times of stress, to lighten the load on your immune system and list for you what nutrient will support and strengthen immunity.

Definition

The immune system is a complex system that depends on the interaction of many different cells, organs and proteins for its optimal function. Its task is to identify and eliminate foreign substances that invade the body and threaten our health. Vital components of the immune system include the thymus glands, bone marrow, lymphatic system, the liver and the spleen.

Symptoms

Indications that the immune system is not functioning at optimal health include chronic respiratory problems, fatigue, allergies, yeast overgrowth, frequent colds and flu, swollen glands, asthma, skin rashes, digestive complaints and frequent headaches.

Dietary considerations

Eat as close to the "original garden" as possible, with plenty of fresh fruits and vegetables, high-fiber foods, seafood, yogurt and kefir. Add garlic and onions to your recipes for added immune-boosting benefit. Avoid sugary foods, which depress immunity (pies, cakes). Avoid fried foods, red meat and refined foods.

Supplement support for the immune system

- B complex
- Olive leaf extract
- Green tea
- Moducare: a plant sterol by Natural Balance
- Bio-K liquid acidophilus
- Power mushrooms: maitake, shiitake and/or reishi
- Astragalus
- Milk thistle extract
- Coenzyme Q$_{10}$: 100 mg daily
- Plant enzymes with each meal
- Raw thymus glandular
- Ester C: 3,000 mg daily
- A daily green drink (Kyo-Green)

Lifestyle choices

- Get enough rest.
- Stop smoking.
- Use massage therapy.
- Start to exercise.
- Get fifteen minutes of early morning sunlight daily.
- Laugh with friends.
- Practice deep breathing.
- Deepen your prayer life.
- Recommended reading: *90-Day Immune System Makeover* by Janet C. Maccaro, Ph.D. (Siloam Press, 2000)

RISKS TO YOUR IMMUNE SYSTEM—WHAT CAN GO WRONG?

Poor diet	According to the *American Journal of Clinical Nutrition,* a study found that sugar slowed the ability of the immune system to eradicate, engulf and consume alien material. Sugar's effect on insulin levels restricts vitamin C's role in allowing immune cells to travel and destroy invaders in our body.[58]
Lack of sleep	Regeneration takes place while you sleep. Rebuilding processes occur during sleep that do not take place during waking hours. Sleep experts agree that while the minimum amount needed for a properly functioning immune system is seven hours of sleep per night, the optimal amount is still eight hours.
Alcohol	Consumption of alcohol lowers immunity by inhibiting the ability of your white cells to react to infections.
Stress	A study reported in *Lancet* showed that blood taken from widows and widowers who were in the grieving process had reduced natural killer cell activity. Stress and a depressed mental outlook can lower immunity.[59]
Overweight	According to the *American Journal of Clinical Nutrition,* eating a low-fat diet may help boost the activity of your natural killer cells, thereby enhancing your immune response.[60]

INSOMNIA

Definition
Insomnia is defined as habitual sleeplessness.

Symptoms
Symptoms include inability to fall asleep, waking during the night and being unable to go back to sleep.

Causes
The causes of insomnia are varied. Anxiety, depression, tension and chronic stress are the most common psychological factors. Physical pain is another cause for insomnia, as well as asthma, hypoglycemia, indigestion, drugs and muscle aches. In addition, if you consume iced tea, coffee or soft drinks that contain sugar and caffeine, you should know that these drinks all contribute to sleepless nights.

Sleep disorders such as snoring or sleep apnea can be serious as they are often linked to irregular heartbeat, high blood pressure and decreased work productivity due to excessive fatigue. Insomnia can be a particularly trouble-some condition because the more you try to fall asleep, the more you cannot. Commercial sleeping pills are not the answer, although they are highly popular these days, because they will interfere with your ability to dream.

Dreaming is your mind's way of getting rid of stored stress. To suppress this natural way to resolve stress is counterproductive. In addition, sleep aids can be habit forming. The chart below shows a protocol that has been used to deal naturally with insomnia, allowing sleep to occur without medication.

Good sleep habits

The following tips about sleeping make sense for all ages:

- Go to bed and awake at the same time each day, even on weekends.
- There is no way to make up for "lost sleep."
- Establish a daily "cool-down" time. One hour before bedtime, dim the lights and eliminate noise. Use this time for low-level stimulation activities such as listening to quiet music or reading nonstimulating material.
- Associate beds with resting only. Talk on the phone or surf the Internet elsewhere.
- Don't drink caffeinated drinks in the afternoon or evening. Caffeine's stimulating effects will peak two to four hours after consumption, but can linger in the body for several hours.
- Don't eat dinner close to bedtime, and don't overeat. Sleep can be disrupted by digestive systems working extra hard after a heavy meal.
- Avoid exercise close to bedtime. Physical activity late in the day can affect your body's ability to relax into a peaceful slumber.

NATURAL SLEEP PROTOCOL

- Before bed take a warm Epsom salts bath with lavender oil added. This will relax your muscles and mind, promoting restful sleep.
- Try some Sleepy Time or Chamomile tea sweetened with Stevia Extract before you go to bed.
- CalMax Powder, which is a highly absorbable calcium-magnesium supplement, will help you sleep through the night.
- Kava and passionflower are natural relaxers, along with valerian root; they help ease tension and cause you to feel sleepy.
- Carbohydrates can also help to induce sleep. Pasta for dinner with vegetables (no meat) is the way to go.
- You may snack on brown rice, bananas or warm milk with honey.
- Do not eat late at night. Make your last meal of the day a light one, and do not consume caffeine late in the day.
- Try 0.3 mg of melatonin on a temporary basis to help reset your biological clock.
- Consider exercise. It is a wonderful stress reliever, which will in turn lighten your mental load.

Health Update — A Natural Tranquilizer

L-theanine (L-T) is the major free-form amino acid found in green tea leaves. L-T produces a tranquilizing effect in the brain without causing drowsiness or dull feelings. Studies reflect that L-T increases alpha waves in the brain that produce muscle relaxation and decrease stress-tension pain.[61] (See L-Theanine: The Antidote to Modern Stress, page 213.)

Bedtime relaxation cocktail: ½ cup water, ½ cup grape juice, one to two capsules of L-theanine opened and poured into the juice, ten to twenty drops of liquid magnesium chloride. Drink this cocktail thirty minutes before bed.

KIDNEY PROBLEMS

Kidney problems can be prevented through improved diet along with herb and supplement therapy.

Definition
Kidney problems include inflammation and/or infection of the kidney(s), sometimes accompanied by kidney stones.

Symptoms
Symptoms include painful frequent urination, chronic lower back pain, fever, fatigue, chills and fluid retention.

Causes
Kidney problems are usually caused by excess sugar, red meat, carbonated drinks and caffeine in the diet; diabetes; allergies; heavy metal poisoning; excess aluminum; EFA deficiency; overuse of prescription drugs; B-vitamin and magnesium deficiency; and overuse of aspirin, salt and diuretics.

Dietary considerations
Have a green drink (Kyo-Green or liquid chlorophyll) every morning. Follow that drink with a low-salt, low-protein, vegetarian diet for at least one month. Avoid all refined, fried and fatty foods as well as soft drinks during the healing phase. Eliminate dairy and animal protein. Drink eight glasses of pure water each day.

Supplement support for kidney problems
To reduce kidney inflammation:

- Quercetin: 1000 mg daily
- Bromelain: 1500 mg daily
- B complex with vitamin B_6
- Magnesium: 800 mg daily
- Flax oil
- Choline/inositol capsules daily

To help reverse kidney damage:

- Gingko biloba
- Enzymedica Purify capsules
- Spirulina capsule: one daily

For infection:

- Cranberry capsules as directed on the bottle
- Biotic Silver
- Echinacea extract as directed on the bottle

Lifestyle choices

- Avoid NSAIDS (Advil, Motrin, Aleve, etc.), which have been associated with impaired kidney function.
- Avoid smoking and secondhand smoke.
- Take a brisk walk every day.
- Apply castor oil packs to kidney area, alternating with ginger packs to stimulate circulation and flow.
- Do not use antacids (Tums, etc.) for indigestion because they may increase the risk of kidney stones.

LIVER PROBLEMS

A healthy liver is truly vital to a healthy, robust life. This is because the health and vitality of every body system depends on the vitality of your liver. Common causes of liver dysfunction include consuming too much alcohol or drugs, sugar, refined foods, preservatives and animal protein. It is triggered as well by low-fiber diets, exposure to toxic chemical and pollutants, stress, candida and chronic sinus infection.

Fortunately, the liver has amazing regenerative powers. It will take six months to a year to regenerate the liver and improve its function. The chart on page 190 gives recommendations that have shown results time and time again.

Definition

Liver problems consist of inflammation and/or infection of the liver.

Symptoms

Symptoms include poor digestion, tiredness, weight gain, sluggish system, depression, food and chemical sensitivities, constipation, nausea, dizziness, jaundiced skin, skin itching and congestion.

Supplement support for liver problems

- Milk thistle seed liquid extract
- Dandelion root extract
- Artichoke capsules
- Reishi or maitake mushroom extract
- Royal jelly
- Germanium: 150 mg
- Bio-K or other acidophilus liquid cultures

- Antioxidants are key, especially coenzyme Q_{10}: 100 mg daily; beta carotene: 10,000 IU daily; and vitamin C (Ester C): 3000 mg daily.
- Keep bowel function optimal: two to three bowel movements daily.

NATURAL PROTOCOL FOR LIVER SUPPORT

- Exercise daily. Your liver is dependent on high-quality oxygen coming into the lungs.
- Drink eight to ten glasses of pure water with lemon each day.
- Keep fats low in your diet.
- Detoxify your body.
- Avoid acid-forming foods (red meat, caffeine, alcohol, dairy products and fried foods).
- Increase potassium-rich foods like seafood and dried fruits.
- Increase chlorophyll-rich foods like leafy greens, and have a green drink daily (Kyo-Green from Wakunaga).
- Increase sulfur-rich foods like eggs, garlic and onions.

LUPUS

This disease is devastating because the immune system becomes disoriented and creates antibodies that attack its own tissue. Joints and connective tissue are especially affected, causing arthritis-like symptoms. The kidneys and lymph nodes become inflamed, along with the heart, brain and central nervous system. For improvement to occur, the immune system must be addressed and toxins must be neutralized. Affecting over half a million Americans, most sufferers are Hispanic or black women (80 percent of all cases).[62]

Definition

Lupus is a multisystem, autoimmune, inflammatory viral disease.

Symptoms

Symptoms include extreme fatigue, low immunity, kidney problems, chronic low-grade fever, arthritis symptoms, photo sensitivity, anemia and red skin patches.

Causes

Viral infections, too many antibiotics or prescription drugs, allergies, emotional stress, reaction to certain chemicals, overgrowth of candida yeast and chronic fatigue syndrome all are causes of lupus.

Dietary considerations

Eat fresh foods, and avoid the nightshade vegetables that may aggravate lupus (tobacco, tomatoes, eggplant and peppers).

Supplement support for lupus

To reduce inflammation, take:

- Quercetin: 1000 mg
- Bromelain: 1500 mg
- MSM capsules: 800 mg

For arthritis symptoms, take:

- Glucosamine: 1500 mg
- Germanium: 150 mg
- L-carnitine: 1000 mg

For stress relief, choose one or more:

- Siberian ginseng extract
- Reishi mushroom extract
- GABA
- SAM-e: 800 mg daily
- Core Level Adrenal
- Kava extract
- Valerian root
- L-theanine

For muscle pain, take:

- Magnesium gel capsules: 400 mg twice daily
- Malic Acid
- B-complex vitamins

To boost immunity, take:

- Astragalus extract
- Royal jelly
- Vitamin C: 3000 mg

For hormone balance:

- Dr. Janet's Balanced by Nature Progesterone Cream

Lifestyle choices

- Take a walk every day for exercise to relieve stress.
- Rest and sleep enough each day.
- Focus on your prayer life.

POWERFUL POTASSIUM DRINK

Have a potassium drink daily. Prepare the following in a juicer:

3 carrots	1 Tbsp. snipped parsley
3 stalks celery	1 tsp. Bragg's Liquid Aminos
½ bunch spinach	

Makes one 12-ounce glass of natural healing nectar.

Menopause

Menopause traditionally occurs in a woman's late forties to early fifties, but it can vary widely between each individual. Many factors influence the timing of menopause, including:

- Trauma, which can trigger premature menopause before age forty because prolonged stress can stop the production of sex hormones.
- Surgery, because if the ovaries are removed, then menopause begins immediately.
- Low body weight, which brings on early menopause due to decreased hormone output by the ovaries. Anorexia can cause them to shut down completely.
- Being overweight, which can delay menopause because extra fat increases estradiol.
- Adrenal exhaustion, caused by too much stress and poor diet, which causes early menopause.

Physically active and well-nourished women experience late menopause while smokers experience earlier menopause.

Definition

Menopause, which means a woman's last menses, is the cessation of menstruation, when the ovaries cease releasing eggs and producing estrogen.

Symptoms

Symptoms include hot flashes, memory loss, depression and irritability, mood swings, anxiety, vaginal dryness and pain, insomnia, low sex drive, night sweats, weight gain, incontinence, inability to focus and concentrate, heart palpitations and nausea.

Dietary considerations

Add soy foods to your diet, and eat fresh vegetables, fruits and nuts. Eat small meals throughout the day instead of three large ones. Limit sugar, caffeine, pies, cakes, pastries, red meat and dairy products.

Supplement support for menopause

- Evening primrose oil: 1,300 mg three times daily
- Black currant seed oil
- Dong quai: high in phytoestrogens
- Red raspberry
- Licorice: adrenal health
- Dr. Janet's Woman's Balance Formula (progesterone cream)
- Black cohosh
- Bioflavonoids: high in phytoestrogens
- Plant enzymes with meals
- Vitamin C
- Dr. Janet's Balanced by Nature Safe Passage Formula
- Vitamin E: hormone normalizer

- B complex
- Raw female glandular
- Adrenal glandular
- 5-HTP: for insomnia and anxiety at night

Lifestyle choices

- Have a bone density test performed to measure bone mass.
- Do weight-bearing exercise.
- Have a regular mammogram. Thermography is a new technique used in conjunction with mammography.
- Enjoy laughter—have a good laugh daily.
- Have massage therapy.
- Practice deep breathing.
- Do Pilates' Exercise, a non-impact series of stretching, strengthening and toning exercises developed by Joseph Pilates.

Natural progesterone cream

Many natural medicine practitioners turn to natural progesterone cream to combat the estrogen dominance syndrome that occurs at the premenopausal and menopausal time of life. Natural progesterone is associated with a feeling of tranquility. Estrogen tends to be irritating to the nervous system if not balanced with progesterone. Balance is the key. Many of the symptoms discussed earlier are the result of high estrogen levels in relationship to progesterone levels.

Phytoestrogens, which are estrogens derived from plant sources, have a beneficial effect on hormonal regulation. Xenoestrogens, which are chemical substances that mimic estrogen when it's stored in body fat, interfere with hormonal regulation and tend to accumulate over time. Because of the accumulation, xenoestrogens are being blamed for diseases ranging from endometriosis, fibroid tumors, ovarian cancer and breast cancer.

Menopause and adrenal health

If you are a woman going through menopause, it is crucial that you attend to the health of your adrenal glands because they help to pick up the slack for your ovaries as their hormone production decreases. Finding an adrenal glandular supplement with licorice and Siberian ginseng in the same formula is especially beneficial to help stimulate the adrenals to regulate body energy and vibrancy during and after menopause.

Menopause: time to reevaluate

Menopause does not signal the end of your vitality, attractiveness and purpose in life. It is a time of reevaluation, a time to focus on the rest of your life. It is an opportunity to accomplish the desires of your heart. It is a time of wisdom and a time for sharing the wisdom and talents that are uniquely yours. Many women experience "postmenopausal zest" for life— and so it should be. It is a wonderful time for self-discovery, service and spiritual maturity.

MENOPAUSE SUGGESTED READING

What Your Doctor May Not Tell You About Menopause by John R. Lee, M.D. (Warner Books)

HRT, Yes or No by Betty Kamen (Nutrition Encounter)

Menopause Without Medicine by Linda Ojeda, Ph.D. (Hunter House Publ.)

The Wisdom of Menopause by Christiane Northrup, M.D. (Bantam Books)

PAIN

Emotional and mental stress can eventually manifest as physical pain. Pain serves to signal us to attend to its underlying cause. Pain dampens your strength and spirit, causing depression.

While painkillers allow you to ignore the pain temporarily so you can work, live and function better, they do nothing to address the cause of the pain. In addition, pain relievers can be addictive or damaging to the stomach lining as well as the liver and kidneys. There are natural methods to overcome pain in the body. They work at a very deep level in the body, relaxing, soothing and calming the area in pain. The following recommendations have been proven to aid in the relief of many different pain syndromes.

Definition
Pain is the physical mechanism the body uses to draw attention to a potential problem.

Symptoms
Symptoms include sharp, shooting twinges or a dull ache, numbness, muscle wasting and poor reflexes.

Causes
Causes of pain include adrenal and pituitary exhaustion, obesity, internal or external tumors, poor nutrition, overly acid diet and poor muscle development, as well as injury and other disease factors.

Dietary considerations
Eat a vegetarian diet, low in fats and high in minerals. Avoid caffeine, sugar and salty foods that create an acidic system. Also, have a green drink each day, such as Kyo-Green by Wakunaga.

Supplements to support pain relief
Herbal pain relievers:

- White willow bark: anti-inflammatory and analgesic
- Kava: relieves stress from chronic pain or injury
- Valerian: a sedative that will help you relax and sleep
- St. John's wort: for nerve damage and to lift the spirits

Other natural pain killers:

- DLPA: 1000 mg daily
- Turmeric
- GABA: 750 mg daily
- Glucosamine capsules and Dr. Janet's Balanced by Nature Glucosamine Cream

Enzymes to reduce inflammation:

- Enzymedica's Purify
- Bromelain
- Quercetin
- MSM
- Boswellia

Lifestyle choices

- Chiropractic adjustments
- Massage therapy
- Therapeutic baths
- Magnet therapy

PREMENSTRUAL SYNDROME (PMS)

Although there are no hard statistics, it is estimated that 70 to 75 percent of American women between the ages of fourteen and fifty suffer from PMS. Five percent have symptoms so severe as to be incapacitating, while 30 to 40 percent report symptoms severe enough to disrupt their daily activities.[63] The good news is that natural remedies are available to balance a woman's body and keep symptoms under control, while at the same time going to the root of the problem.

Stress is a huge trigger of PMS because it impacts both estrogen and progesterone levels. In addition, stress increases the occurrence of intestinal yeast, which produces estrogen-like substances. When a woman is under stress, her progesterone levels plummet because progesterone converts into adrenal hormones to meet the demands of the overworked adrenal glands, thus creating the hormonal imbalance that contributes to PMS.

Definition

PMS (premenstrual syndrome) is related to hormonal imbalance, involving the ratio of estrogen to progesterone. PMS results from inadequate levels of progesterone in the second half of the menstrual cycle. This creates an "estrogen dominant" situation, which results in blood sugar irregularities, depression, water retention and more.

Estrogen dominance occurs more often in women these days because of xenoestrogens (foreign estrogens) from environmental pollutants like pesticides, plastic-lined cans and so forth. In addition, beef, poultry and milk products are laden with growth hormones that can contribute to estrogen dominance. Stress lowers progesterone levels, leaving women vulnerable to estrogen dominance.

Symptoms

Symptoms of PMS include low back pain, fatigue, breast tenderness, bloating, irritability, carbohydrate cravings, cramps, constipation, irregular periods, skin eruptions, depression and anxiety. These symptoms occur during the second half of the menstrual cycle and intensify during the week just before the onset of a period.

Dietary considerations

Buy organic meat, milk and milk products and organic canned foods to avoid chemicals that create xenoestrogens. Eat dark leafy greens and whole grains. Add soy and flaxseed, or other sources of essential fatty acids, to your diet.

Supplement support for PMS

PMS sufferers have been grouped into four categories according to their symptoms by Guy A. Abraham, M.D., but some physicians have gone so far as to add a fifth category that includes painful periods, cramps, low back pain, nausea and vomiting.[64] Specific supplementation is helpful to each different set of symptoms. (See page 197.)

Homeopathic helps

For low back pain or cramps, take five pellets of the following at the onset of pain, and repeat every fifteen minutes until symptoms abate:

- ❦ Cimicifuga: 12C
- ❦ Magnesia Phosphorica: 12C
- ❦ Nux Vomica: 12C

For depression, irritability and water retention, take five pellets in the morning of Sepia, 12C, and Lac Caninum, 12C. Take five pellets in the evening of Folliculnum, 12C.[65]

PMS CATEGORIES

Type A—Anxiety	Characterized by emotional symptoms including anxiety, irritability and mood swings	Magnesium: 400–600 mg Calcium: 800–1200 mg B complex: 1 capsule Passionflower Valerian GABA Dr. Janet's Woman's Balance Formula, a transdermal cream
Type C—Cravings	Characterized by cravings for simple carbohydrates like breads, sugary foods, chips, etc., resulting in blood sugar imbalances with peaks and valleys; fatigue, dizziness and headaches	Eat small meals throughout the day. B complex: 50–100 mg of each B vitamin Chromium picolinate: 200 mcg daily (400 mcg. if over 150 pounds) Calcium: 800–1,200 mg Magnesium: 400–800 mg Dr. Janet's Woman's Balance Formula, a transdermal cream
Type D—Depression	Characterized by withdrawal from normal daily activities, insomnia, sadness, crying and confusion	5-HTP: as directed on bottle B complex: 100 mg of each of the B vitamins Magnesium: 400–800 mg Calcium: 800–1,200 mg. Sleep Link: for insomnia Dr. Janet's Woman's Balance Formula, a transdermal cream
Type H—Hyperhydration	Characterized by water retention, bloating, weight gain, breast tenderness and swelling	B complex: one capsule twice daily Magnesium: 200–600 mg Vitamin E: 400–800 IU Evening primrose oil: 1,500 mg Calcium: 800–1,200 mg Potassium: 1–2 gm Dr. Janet's Woman's Balance Formula, a transdermal cream
Type P—Pain	Characterized by low back pain, nausea, vomiting, cramps and painful periods	Vitamin B_6: 100–300 mg B complex: 50–100 mg of each of the B vitamins Magnesium: 400–800 mg Evening primrose oil Calcium: 800–1,200 mg Vitamin E: 400–800 IU Dr. Janet's Woman's Balance Formula, a transdermal cream

PROSTATE HEALTH

Definition
Benign prostate hyperplasia (BPH) is common in men over the age of fifty.

Symptoms
Symptoms include nocturnal urination and restricted flow due to enlarged prostate gland. This may be related to a change or reduction in the metabolism of testosterone.
SEE ANDROPAUSE

RHEUMATIC FEVER

This condition primarily affects children before they become teens. Rheumatic fever can be prevented if a strep infection is treated in time (within ten to twelve days of initial infection). If rheumatic fever is contracted, it tends to recur, affecting the heart, brain and joints and producing arthritis-like symptoms. Natural medicine concentrates on building the immune system to the highest possible level to prevent future illness since the main cause is low immunity.

Definition
Rheumatic fever is a serious inflammatory illness that usually follows a strep infection.

Symptoms
Symptoms of rheumatic fever include skin rash, shortness of breath, sore throat, poor circulation, fever and extreme fatigue and weakness. Arthritis is the most common symptom, often lasting a lifetime.

Dietary considerations
Eat fresh foods, and drink fresh fruit and vegetable juices. Avoid sugar, refined foods, fried foods, caffeine and soft drinks. Drink eight to ten glasses of spring water daily.

Supplement support for rheumatic fever

- After antibiotic therapy, Kyo-Dophilus or Bio-K liquid acidophilus
- Coenzyme Q_{10}: 100 mg daily for heart strength
- Kyolic Garlic capsules
- Carlson's ACES: antioxidant protection
- Ascorbate vitamin C: 3,000–5,000 mg daily
- Daily green drink (Kyo-Green): to strengthen immunity
- Dr. Janet's Glucosamine Cream: to ease arthritis symptoms
- Refer to my book *90-Day Immune System Makeover* to rebuild immunity.

Lifestyle choices

- ❦ Make sure to rest properly.
- ❦ Take sea salt and baking soda baths.
- ❦ Get massage therapy.
- ❦ Practice deep breathing.
- ❦ Alert all physicians to your condition, especially your dentist. You may need antibiotic medication before dental procedures.

SCIATICA

The pain that sciatica causes can be excruciating, making the quality of life extremely poor. Causes include poor posture, obesity, poor spinal alignment, not drinking enough water, improper lifting, stress, nutrient deficiency and poor abdominal tone. The good news is that help is available, help that is safe and natural and addresses not just the pain, but also the root cause.

Definition

Sciatica is pain along the sciatic nerve that radiates down the back of the leg.

Symptoms

Symptoms include lower back pain and severe pain in the leg along the course of the sciatic nerve that usually begins at the back of the thigh and runs down the inside of the leg.

Dietary considerations

Eat a diet low in fat and high in vegetables, protein and minerals. Drink six to eight glasses of water daily. Avoid caffeine, sugar, red meat and dairy. Have a whey protein shake each morning.

Supplement support for sciatica

- ❦ Dr. Janet's Glucosamine Cream (with emu oil, pregnenolone, glucos-amine, boswellia, bromelain, MSM): use as needed on affected area
- ❦ DLPA: 1,000 mg
- ❦ MSM: 1,000 mg
- ❦ Glucosamine sulfate: 1,000–1,500 mg
- ❦ Vitamin C: 3,000 mg
- ❦ Magnesium chloride liquid: ten to fifteen drops at bedtime
- ❦ Daily green drink (Kyo-Green)

Lifestyle choices

- ❦ Manage your stress.
- ❦ Use warm castor oil packs.
- ❦ Strengthen abdominal muscles.
- ❦ Exercise regularly.
- ❦ Buy a firm mattress.
- ❦ Use massage therapy.
- ❦ Get chiropractic treatments.

Shingles

Definition
Shingles is an acute inflammation of the nerves caused by the *Vericella-Zoster* virus, accompanied by pain and burning over small or large parts of the body

Symptoms
Fever and chills precede the attack. Then blisters develop around the upper part of the body, after which painful nerves remain irritated for several weeks. Areas affected include hands, neck, face, chest, limbs and especially the rib area.

Initially, there is an itching or sensitivity in the area of attack, followed by a rash with small raised spots that turn into blisters. These blisters are filled with viral organisms. They are very itchy and extremely painful, often feeling like severe burns. The blisters dry out and leave scabs that eventually fall off, leaving behind scars. Unfortunately, this is not the end of the attack. The pain that lingers can be severe and last for months or even years because it is caused by nerve damage. Shingles that occur on the face or eye area are far more serious because of the possibility of blindness or facial paralysis.

Causes
Chronic or prolonged periods of stress compromise immunity, thus allowing the *Vericella-Zoster* virus (which causes chicken pox) to reemerge as shingles. Other triggers include physical stress to the point of exhaustion, lymphoma, Hodgkin's disease and anticancer drugs.

Dietary considerations
Consider a juicing program for three to five days, followed by eating plenty of fresh vegetables and fruit. Avoid immune-suppressing substances: sugar, caffeine, alcohol, white flour, nicotine and animal fats. Add fiber to your diet, and drink plenty of water.

Supplement support for shingles
- L-lysine: inhibits the spread of the disease
- Vitamin B_{12}: promotes healing
- St. John's wort: antiviral
- Beta carotene: enhances immunity
- Vitamin E: promotes healing
- Echinacea: boosts immunity and has antiviral properties
- Pau d'arco: cleanses the blood and strengthens the liver
- Dr. Janet's Balanced by Nature Glucosamine Cream
- Reishi, maitake and shiitake mushrooms: boost immunity
- Passionflower: calms the nerves
- Hops: calms the nerves
- Valerian root: calms the nerves
- Daily green drink

Lifestyle choices

- ❧ Ice packs can be used to cool and soothe an infected area.
- ❧ Avoid further stress.
- ❧ Listen to peaceful music.
- ❧ Practice deep breathing.
- ❧ Take long walks in the early morning.
- ❧ Get plenty of rest.
- ❧ Have weekly or monthly massage therapy.
- ❧ Polysporin can help prevent infection.

SINUSITIS

One in three Americans suffer from a chronic sinus infection.[66] The physical causes vary, including allergies; too much dairy, sugar, salt and fried foods; poor food combining; constipation; poor circulation; and a bacterial, fungal or viral infection. This is a very uncomfortable condition that leaves the sufferer feeling worn out, tired and with a postnasal drip that makes it especially hard to sleep.

Definition

Sinusitis is an inflammation of the sinuses with labored breathing.

Symptoms

Symptoms include inflamed nasal passages, postnasal drip, sore throat, facial pain, loss of smell and taste, pressure headaches around the sinus, bad breath, indigestion, earaches and toothaches. There may be nausea and indigestion from swallowed mucus as well.

Dietary considerations

Drink plenty of fresh juices (pineapple and grape are especially good). Eliminate wheat and dairy products, and avoid alcoholic beverages. Sipping hot herbal teas can help initiate mucus flow. Using horseradish on food helps to clear the sinuses.

Supplement support for sinusitis

- ❧ Detoxification with Nature's Secret Ultimate Cleanse
- ❧ To address the infection: Biotic Silver, grapefruit seed extract capsules or olive leaf extract capsules, and nasal spray
- ❧ For congestion: Breathe Easy tea from Traditional Medicinals; Ester C, 3,000 mg daily; echinacea extract, fifteen drops in water four times daily
- ❧ To boost immunity: astragalus capsules; B complex with pantothenic acid; Kyolic Garlic capsules as directed

Keep in mind that over-the-counter drug store sinus medications only suppress symptoms and may drive the infection deeper into the sinus cavities. Natural medicine goes to the root cause.

It is imperative that you build up your immune system. Please read my book *90-Day Immune System Makeover,* which I refer to several times in this book.

SKIN HEALTH

Beautiful skin comes naturally in our youth. When we are young, our skin is soft, supple and glowing. But as we age, beautiful skin is a reward for taking proper care of our bodies. The skin is a barometer, which reflects what is going on with us internally.

Skin care is big business these days as baby boomers anxiously take part in staving off the signs of aging. Stress, excessive sun exposure, liver malfunction, hormone depletion, smoking, alcohol, sugar, fried foods, caffeine and poor circulation all contribute to the deterioration of our skin. Age spots, wrinkles, dry skin, uneven skin tone, sallow complexion and acne are the result of how well our systems handle wastes. Free-radical damage is also a major contributor to poor skin.

Definition
Skin health can be defined as the care to maintain healthy skin.

Health Update	Beauty Big Three

Detoxify and eat healthy.
Moisturize and drink plenty of water.
Protect by limiting sun exposure and using sunscreen.

Dietary considerations
Eat fresh fruit and vegetables each day. Fruits are wonderful cleansers. Drink eight to ten glasses of water daily, and add fresh lemon for cleansing. Make a fresh "liver cocktail" each day from fresh juice that consists of 2 ounces beet juice, 3 ounces of carrot juice and 3 ounces of cucumber juice. (Use a juicer.) Avoid sugar, caffeine and red meat to prevent dehydration.

Supplement support for healthy skin

- Nature's Secret Ultimate Cleanse and liver flush (page 223)
- Gingko biloba: to increase circulation
- Carlson's ACES: for free-radical damage
- Coenzyme Q_{10}: 100 mg daily
- Evening primrose oil
- Dr. Janet's Woman's Balance Progesterone Formula
- Dr. Janet's Balanced by Nature SkinTastic
- Dr. Janet's Balanced by Nature Skin Cream

Lifestyle choices

- Reduce or prevent wrinkles by rubbing papaya skins on the face.

(Papain is an enzyme that exfoliates the skin.)

- Use alpha-hydroxy acids (fruit acid) to exfoliate the skin.
- Manage stress.
- Practice deep breathing.
- Have a massage with almond oil, sesame oil or wheat germ oil to soften the skin.
- Moisturize immediately after bathing.
- Rub lemon juice on age spots, or use 2 percent hydroquinone topical cream to reduce and fade age spots.
- Limit sun exposure. Always use a sunblock SPF-15 or more to prevent further damage and to prevent age spots from darkening.

Health Update — Helping Your Skin

- Watermelon

Watermelon juice is rich in natural silica, which supports collagen and reduces wrinkled and dry skin.

- Detox signal

The condition of your skin can be the first thing to alert you that you need to start a detoxification program. If your colon becomes stagnant with toxins and your liver does not filter wastes and impurities coming from the digestive tract, your skin will give you one or more of many sure signs—rashes, acne, boils, blotchiness, uneven skin tone, dermatitis and itchy skin. After detoxification, your skin will glow, and your skin problems will diminish or disappear.

SMOKING

Everyone knows that smoking is hazardous to your health. After all, we are living in the information age. And since we are, let me give you a little more information about smoking that you may not be aware of. Smoking is the largest single preventable cause of illness and premature death in the United States.[67] It is connected to chronic bronchitis and emphysema, cancers of the lung, larynx, pharynx, mouth, esophagus, pancreas and bladder. There is also a connection linking smoking during pregnancy with complications and retarded fetal development. In addition, smoking ages you. According to the Canadian Cancer Society, a one-pack-a-day smoker is physically as old at age fifty as a nonsmoker at age fifty-eight![68]

My own father was a smoker. I can remember him going for a bicycle ride after dinner while smoking a cigarette! You should also know my father suffered from heart disease, emphysema and cancer. You know that the health hazards of smoking are numerous, including endangering your loved ones, especially children, because of the dangerous effect of secondhand smoke. You are predisposing your family or coworkers to respiratory illness or possibly nicotine-related cancer. If you do not stop smoking for benefits to yourself, then do it for those around you. It is a dangerous, expensive and dirty habit that stains your hands and teeth and fouls your breath. It pollutes your home, car and workplace. Before your smoking habit kills you, kill your smoking habit.

Fourteen-day plan to quit smoking

I realize that quitting the smoking habit can be one of the hardest tasks that you ever undertake. But when you are ready, I have a plan to help you kick the habit and reverse the damage that has already occurred. That's the good news. It is encouraging to know that almost all of the health hazards can be totally reversed once you stop smoking. Here is how the plan works.

First, make sure that you begin on the weekend, ideally, Saturday. Do not begin while you are on vacation or under unusual stress from your job. Try to begin this plan when you are on a regular schedule and during a relatively calm time of the year. Avoid seasons of parties, birthdays, tax time and so forth.

Second, mark a goal on your calendar. Label that day "Smoke Free!" Then begin to work toward that goal. You should be able to accomplish your goal of being smoke free in about fourteen days. While some people achieve their goal sooner, I have found that the fourteen-day plan works for most of my clients. To achieve your goal of becoming smoke free, follow the steps outlined in the chart below.

FOURTEEN-DAY PLAN TO QUIT SMOKING

1. During the first seven days, be sure to eat as close to nature as possible—no processed or refined foods.
2. Take 200 mg of chromium. If you are over 150 pounds, take 400 mcg.
3. Cut the number of cigarettes you smoke this first week by one-half. Chromium will help to balance your blood sugar, thereby lessening any symptoms of withdrawal. If you feel the urge to smoke, just chew gum or munch on carrot or celery sticks to satisfy the feeling of having to have something in your mouth.
4. Get rid of all lighters and matches. Tell your family, friends and coworkers that you are giving up this health-destroying habit, and enlist their support.
5. On the eighth day, cut your smoking by half once again. You may experience withdrawal symptoms. Some people are fortunate and do not have withdrawal symptoms. The majority of people, however, do suffer from very mild to very difficult withdrawal symptoms, which may include headache, tiredness, cough, nervousness, dizziness, constipation, sore throat and craving for a cigarette. All of these symptoms are temporary.

6. To help minimize withdrawal symptoms, try exercising, sleeping more at night, drinking plenty of water and eating a lot of fresh fruit to help even out the release of nicotine from the body. If you are constipated, slowly add fiber to your diet, and this problem should pass quickly. Just be patient and ride out these symptoms. They will pass.
7. On days ten through thirteen continue to cut your cigarettes by one-half each day. By day fourteen you should be smoke free!

Now that you have accomplished this wonderful milestone, ask God to continue to give you strength to move forward into your smoke-free environment, never backward. Cigarette smoking is now in your past. Take a deep breath, and know that each breath you take from this moment on is helping regenerate your entire body. Keep taking the chromium; it will help you conquer any unhealthy cravings, whether for cigarettes, sugar or alcohol.

After you break the smoking habit, get your car cleaned and detailed to rid the smell of smoke; clean your house from top to bottom, washing drapes, rugs, walls and counters; throw away ash trays. Keep chewing gum handy when you're under stress, and always remember how wonderful it is to be set free from smoking.

Homeopathic remedies
Use Nico-Stop by Enzymatic Therapy or Nico-End by Phytopharmica to reduce the craving for nicotine. Take one tablet three times daily and during cravings. Avoid food or drink for ½ hour before or after chewing it. Use for three months for best results. For more information, visit their website at www.enzy.com.

SPORTS INJURIES

Many Americans are "weekend warriors," saving all of their exercise time or yard work for the weekends. While it may be the most convenient or the only time you can squeeze these activities in, this is how most sports injuries occur. Tennis elbow, torn ligaments, bruises, twisted ankles, sprains, shin splints, cramps and more send people to the doctor in pain. Causes also include poor circulation, mineral deficiency, too much fat and sugar in the diet and an over-acidic system. A sprain is caused by a twisting motion that actually causes a tear in the ligaments that secure the joints. Tendonitis is an inflammation of a tendon and usually results from a strain or overexertion. Both conditions are painful and require time and care for proper healing.

Definition
Sports injuries involve muscle pain, tendonitis, sprains and torn ligaments.

Dietary considerations

Consume vegetable protein to speed healing. Add magnesium-rich foods to help relax muscles, such as nuts, beans and whole grains. Have a glass of pineapple juice since bromelain is an anti-inflammatory agent. Avoid sugar, caffeine, red meat and soft drinks during the healing phase. Drink plenty of water to flush toxins.

Supplement support for sports injuries

- Dr. Janet's Glucosamine Cream
- Arnica, for sprains and bruises
- Ruta Graveolens, for pulled tendons
- Rus Tox, for swelling
- Sportenine, for tendonitis
- Magnesium: 800 mg
- B-complex vitamin
- Kava
- L-theanine
- Creatine: 1,000 mg
- Chromium picolinate: 200 mcg
- Vitamin C: 3,000–5,000 mg
- Quercetin
- Bromelain
- Glucosamine: 1,500 mg
- Chondroitin: 1,200 mg
- Silica
- Daily green drink

Lifestyle choices

- Massage area frequently to stimulate circulation.
- Apply ice packs on day of injury: thirty minutes on, fifteen minutes off for the first three to four hours, then alternate between hot and cold packs the following day.
- Be sure to elevate the injury to inhibit swelling.
- Wrap with an Ace bandage if possible to prevent swelling.
- Take a very warm sea salt bath with a few drops of lavender essential oil for stress relief.
- Time is a great healer, giving opportunity for the body to heal itself.

STREP/SORE THROAT

Definition

Strep or sore throat is a symptom that is associated with a viral or bacterial infection in the upper respiratory tract.

SEE PROTOCOL FOR RHEUMATIC FEVER

Health Update	Sore Throat Relief

- To soothe a sore throat, drink a cup of tea made from slippery elm.
- Ginger tea is also effective. Simmer three to four slices of fresh ginger in a cup of water for six to eight minutes.
- Slippery elm lozenges are also available.

STRESS

No matter what your present state of health is, whether you are suffering from stress, fibromyalgia, panic attacks, muscle tension, lupus, chronic fatigue or depression, it is important to remember that it took many years and many life events to bring you to your current level of health. The good news is, though you may feel defeated, you do still have a level of health. And you can begin to initiate some healthful choices that will improve your health for years to come. God desires to help you and is guiding you even as you read this book. I believe God allows us to advance spiritually through adversity.

So, where do we begin? Since you may be feeling overwhelmed by your life or your poor health, I will not overwhelm you with too much technical information. Rather, my goal is to gently educate you and guide you back to a course that will bring you to health. You may be surprised to see how much better you feel just by understanding *why you feel the way you do.*

It has been said that stress is one of the leading causes of doctors' visits in America. With this in mind, I offer you this special section on stress. The following information is a blueprint for building your body and brain back after years of stored trauma and stress.

Definition

Stress is any factor that threatens the body's health, such as injury, worry, disease or toxic chemicals.

Symptoms

When your emotional pain becomes full-fledged anxiety, you may experience any of the symptoms listed in the following chart.

THE BODY-MIND CONNECTION

- Fatigue
- Muscle tension
- Strange aches and pains
- Migraine headaches
- Hot and cold flashes
- Nausea
- Racing heart
- Disorientation
- Panic attacks
- Sweats
- Dizziness
- Scary thoughts
- Depression

Causes

The most common causes of stress are emotional and/or physical problems; work addiction; lack of sleep; ingesting too much sugar, caffeine and alcohol; vitamin and mineral depletion from a poor diet; unemployment; marital problems; being a caregiver and hypoglycemia.

Recognizing the early signs of stress and taking action early on to handle it through exercise, relaxation, dietary changes and prayer, rather than letting stress become destructive, will make a difference in your quality of life and well-being. First, let's find out just how much emotional stress and pain are contributing to your current state of health. There are common backgrounds and personality traits in people who suffer from anxiety and chronic illness. By taking the test below, developed by the Midwest Center for Stress and Anxiety, you can identify some of the stress triggers that you need to address.[69]

STRESS TRIGGERS

CHILDHOOD BACKGROUND

Check the ones that apply to you:

- ❏ Unstable upbringing/divorce of parent
- ❏ Lack of approval and praise
- ❏ Feeling that you must prove yourself as a child
- ❏ Strict religious upbringing/guilt and fear
- ❏ Siblings parenting other siblings
- ❏ Nervous disorders in family
- ❏ Separation or loss of a family member
- ❏ Strict parents with high expectations
- ❏ Family history of alcoholism
- ❏ Low self-esteem
- ❏ Feelings not easily shown or displayed

PERSONALITY TRAITS

Check the ones with which you can identify:

- ❏ Tendency to overreact
- ❏ Perfectionist
- ❏ Inner nervousness
- ❏ Emotionally sensitive
- ❏ Guilt ridden
- ❏ Extremely analytical
- ❏ Overly concerned about others' opinions of you
- ❏ Obsessive thinker
- ❏ Worry about health problems
- ❏ High expectations
- ❏ Inability to make decisions

Now, let's look at the four levels of stress indicated by your reactions to life.[70] This will help you to determine to what level your stress has affected you. Which of these symptoms best fit your daily experience at present?

STRESS LEVELS	
Level I	Losing interest in enjoyable activities Sagging of the corners of the eyes Creasing of the forehead Becoming short tempered Bored, nervous
Level II	All of Level I, plus Tiredness Anger Insomnia Paranoia Sadness
Level III	All of Levels I and II, plus Chronic head and neck aches High blood pressure Upset stomach Looking older
Level IV	All of Levels I, II and III, plus Skin disorders Kidney malfunction Frequent infections Asthma Heart disease Mental or emotional breakdown

Dietary considerations

Besides choosing healthy foods, make mealtimes a pleasant social encounter. Celebrate family time by making menu planning, table setting and cooking together family activities.

To lower stress levels it will be necessary to eliminate sugar, caffeine and soft drinks. These substances tax the adrenal glands and leave them unable to function optimally, resulting in greater stress levels.

Supplement support for stress

For descriptions and instructions for taking the listed amino acids and herbs, see Appendices B and C. For natural protocol for stress, see Appendix D.

- Amino acids: lysine, glutamine, GABA, tyrosine, glycine and taurine
- Siberian ginseng
- Valerian

- ❧ Passionflower
- ❧ St. John's wort
- ❧ Kava
- ❧ 5-HTP
- ❧ For adrenal health: Take pantothenic acid, B complex, vitamin C, royal jelly and astragalus; add dietary recommendations listed in the adrenal section.
- ❧ For hormonal help: Use Dr. Janet's Balanced by Nature Progesterone Cream, and/or Dr. Janet's Balanced by Nature Safe Passage.
- ❧ Dr. Janet's Balanced by Nature Tranquility

Lifestyle choices

- ❧ See Appendix E: Tips for Beating Stress.
- ❧ Massage: Consider having a weekly massage. It will help your muscles relax, thereby relieving tension.
- ❧ Exercise: Begin to exercise; find ways to move. This is one of the best stress relievers in the world. The more you exercise, the more energy you will have.
- ❧ Mantle technique: My "MANTLE Technique" is simply tensing and holding, for the count of ten, each part of your body, one section at a time. (See page 231.)
- ❧ Stress-relieving bath: This should be used periodically to keep your acid alkaline level in balance. (See pages 25 and 64.)
- ❧ Prayer: Develop a life of meaningful communication with your loving God.
- ❧ Bach Essences: Choose the ones that suit your current situation. (See page 53.)

Thank God for GABA

Because of the potential impact the amino acid GABA has proven to have in the relief of severe stress symptoms, I am including a detailed discussion to help you understand how it can help you.

During my lowest point of poor health, I used GABA to replenish my brain. Its effect was truly amazing, calming my mind and body. With my GABA receptors replenished, the false alarms or overfiring stopped and the panic attacks ended. I began to recommend it to my clients who continued to have mind and body symptoms long after they completed their nutritional programs. The results were no less than remarkable. GABA proved to be invaluable in the quest for emotional balance and freedom from anxiety and stress-related illness.

Of all the neurotransmitters in the brain, the amino acid GABA is the most widely distributed in the body. According to Michael J. Gitlin, M.D., it has a very important part to play in the regulation of anxiety.[71] This is because the GABA receptors in the area of the brain that control anxiety became replenished and restored after supplementation with this simple amino acid. Taking this simple amino acid to replenish your brain has no risks or side effects.

GABA is the main inhibitory neurotransmitter that restores the brain. Its function is to regulate anxiety, muscle spasms, depression and chronic stress.

Traumatic memories can be stored throughout your body. Your brain is not the only organ that suffers. Your stomach, skin, muscles, heart, skeletal system and any other organ of your body suffer as well. Since there are GABA receptors throughout your entire body, it is believed that taking GABA in the proper amounts can reduce the stress, anxiety and tension in any of the abovementioned areas of the body.

Many of my clients who complain of stomach trouble almost always have a stress or trauma connection that is unresolved. It is interesting to note that according to Dr. Billie J. Sahley's research, the gut's brain is located in the lining of the stomach, esophagus, small intestine and the colon. The brain in your head communicates with the brain in your gut. Here comes the mind-body connection once more.[72]

Dr. Michael Gershon, a professor of anatomy and cell biology, reported that many gastrointestinal disorders like colitis, irritable bowel syndrome and diverticulitis can originate from problems within the gut's brain.[73] In essence, diarrhea, nausea or constipation, which are common complaints these days, can be a result of prolonged anxiety, stress or emotional pain. This is because the brain in your head communicates with the brain in your gut by way of the neurotransmitters.

GABA is normally in abundant supply throughout the complex network of the mind and body. So when the GABA supply is deficient, both brains suffer, and your body is flooded with uncomfortable, life-disrupting symptoms. It is very possible that your present behavior, state of mind or physical health is a direct result of your stress levels, anxiety, grief, anger, unresolved conflict and resultant deficient GABA.

Effects of GABA depletion

The following chart will show you just how much of an impact anxiety and trauma, both past and present, can have in depleting your GABA supply. This depletion will in turn start a chain reaction of stress-related body symptoms.

TRAUMA DEPLETES GABA

Emotions that deplete GABA:

❧ Pain	❧ Anxiety	❧ Grief
❧ Fear	❧ Anger	❧ Panic

These unresolved emotions lead to:

❧ Chronic pain	❧ Back pain	❧ Neck pain
❧ Illness	❧ Rapid heartbeat	❧ Difficulty breathing
❧ Panic attacks	❧ Insomnia	❧ Headaches
❧ Crying		

GABA depletion affects the entire body.

- Eyes: pupils dilate, blurred vision.
- Mouth: dry mouth, choking sensation
- Heart: racing, palpitations, pounding
- Lungs: difficulty breathing, bronchioles constrict
- Stomach: contracts, nausea, indigestion
- Adrenal glands: release adrenaline rushes, weakness, no energy
- Colon: gas, constipation, diarrhea
- Bladder: frequent urination

Stress and magnesium deficiency

There are other nutrients that work along with GABA for its proper metabolism. One important nutrient is magnesium. Magnesium enhances GABA's action and effect on the body. Interestingly enough, most people with long-standing anxiety and stress problems are deficient in magnesium. Furthermore, it is important to note that the symptoms of magnesium deficiency are the same as those that occur with anxiety, stress and emotional depletion. I have listed for you the symptoms of magnesium deficiency. Compare them to the chart that lists stress and anxiety symptoms, and you will see a very real connection.

SYMPTOMS OF MAGNESIUM DEFICIENCY	
Depression	Dizziness
Muscle spasms	Headaches
Anxiety	Constipation
Panic attacks	Irritable bowel syndrome
Mitral valve prolapse	Asthma
Fibromyalgia	Spastic symptoms
Fatigue	Chronic pain
Low blood sugar	Noise sensitivity
Irregular heartbeat	

Do you see the connection to stress and anxiety symptoms? According to many different experts, simple GABA replenishment can replace some of the most overprescribed medications of our day, such as Prozac, Xanax, Valium and other similar mood-altering drugs. Taken with magnesium, the calming effects are enhanced even more. For me, this was life-changing information. Throughout the years that I suffered physical illness and anxiety symptoms, I always believed that the answer to my condition would come. Thanks to the pioneer in amino acid GABA research, Dr. Candace Pert, it did!

When stress shatters, magnesium saves.

It is likely that depletion of magnesium among type A individuals (competitive behavior, heart disease prone) is the main reason why they are at increased risk of heart attacks. When a person has a heart attack, one of the first things that is administered is magnesium.

Because I am your typical A-type personality, have a family history of heart disease and have experienced stress to the max, I have made magnesium a very important part of my daily dietary supplement protocol. Magnesium taken by mouth is very safe, except if you suffer from kidney disease or if you are severely dehydrated. In that case you could develop levels of magnesium in the blood that are simply too high. Check with your healthcare provider if you are in doubt.

Also, taking too much magnesium may cause drowsiness and lethargy. I personally take and recommend 400 milligrams of magnesium at bedtime. I prefer a gel capsule to a hard tablet. I wholeheartedly recommend supplementation because we Americans consume diets that fail to even meet the government's recommended dietary allowance for magnesium. Most troubling is the fact that among people who develop heart disease, their intake is even lower than average.[74] Because magnesium is the most critical mineral of all for coping with stress, you should, in addition to taking a magnesium supplement, add the following magnesium-rich foods to your diet.

Soybeans	Green beans	Black-eyed peas
Broccoli	Dates	Blackberries
Bananas	Millet	Navy beans
Kidney beans	Kasha (buckwheat)	Almonds
Watermelon	Shrimp	Tuna

Health Update — L-Theanine: The Antidote to Modern Stress

Theanine is an amino acid found in green tea that produces tranquilizing effects in the brain. In Japan, soft drinks and chewing gum are spiked with theanine for the purpose of inducing relaxation.

Although theanine creates a feeling of relaxation, it doesn't shut down the brain. Studies on rodents show that theanine enhances the ability to learn and remember. By shutting off worry central, theanine appears to increase concentration and focus thought.

Theanine is different from kava in that it doesn't cause drowsiness, just relaxation. Theanine increases GABA, while caffeine decreases it. GABA doesn't just relax; it also creates a sense of well-being. Theanine's ability to increase GABA can literally put you in a better mood. Theanine also increases levels of dopamine, another brain chemical with mood-enhancing effects.

The suggested dose of theanine to induce a state of relaxation is 100–400 milligrams daily.

Tumors

Definition

A tumor is a growing lump or nodule attached to the body, malignant or benign.

SEE CYSTS AND POLYPS

Warts

Usually harmless, but very unsightly, warts can be clustered or single in appearance. They are found on the feet, hands, face and arms and can range in size from a speck to a kidney bean. Because they are caused by human papilloma viruses, they can be contagious and will spread if picked at, bitten or cut. Most common warts disappear within a year or two without any treatment. However, the following are recommendations to help prevent their occurrence or shorten the duration.

Definition

A wart is defined as any small growth on the skin associated with a viral infection.

Symptoms

Symptoms are raised or flat growths on the skin surface.

Dietary considerations

Eat as close to the "original garden" as possible. That means eating immune-boosting foods: fresh vegetables and fruits. Include citrus fruits and broccoli. Add sulphur foods like garlic, onions and eggs to your diet. Avoid sugary foods, pies, cakes, candy, soft drinks and processed and refined foods.

Supplement support for warts

- B complex for normal cell multiplication
- Vitamin C: 5,000 mg daily for antiviral effect
- Vitamin A (emulsion form): 100,000 IU daily for one month. The second month use 50,000 IU daily, and the third month graduate down to 25,000 IU until wart is gone.
- Vitamin E: apply topically
- N-acetyl cysteine: 2,000 mg daily for immune response
- Daily green drink (Kyo-Green)

Lifestyle choices

- Do not squeeze, cut, pick or bite at a wart. It can spread or become infected.
- Apply Lysine topical cream.
- Apply lemon juice/sea salt or the inside of papaya skins to wart areas.

❧   Banana Cure: Rub the inside section of a banana peel over the
    wart. Then cut a piece of the inside peel into a square and place it
    over the wart. Secure it with a Band-Aid. Repeat daily until the
    wart is gone. (This "cure" worked for me as a child.)

WEIGHT CONTROL/OBESITY

By definition, half of the population of North America is overweight. One in
every five men and one in every three women in America are considered
obese. Furthermore, one in every four American children is overweight.
Considering these statistics, obesity is an American epidemic.[75]

The good news is that there are safe, effective, natural substances that can
boost the metabolism, decrease the appetite and give you pure energy.
Surgical options always carry high risks and side effects, and caloric restriction is not always healthy. I encourage you to consider the natural options if
you are overweight.

Definition
Overweight is defined as body weight of 20 percent over the normal prescribed weight for a particular age, build or height.

Causes
It is a complex and frustrating problem that has many causative factors:
genetics, lack of exercise, overeating, stress, boredom, low-fiber, high-
carbohydrate diet, glandular and hormonal disorders as well as age-related
metabolic slowdown.

Dietary considerations
A high-fiber diet is essential because fiber improves the excretion of fat,
improves glucose tolerance and gives you a feeling of fullness and satisfaction. Emphasize the following foods: brown rice, tuna, chicken, white fish,
fresh fruits and vegetables, high-protein lean foods, lentils, beans, whole-
grain bread and turkey.

Eat several small meals daily instead of skipping meals and eating one big
meal daily. You want to give your body even-burning fuel throughout the day.
Otherwise, your body will store fat instead of burn it for "survival."

Avoid sugars and snack foods that contain salt and fat, like potato chips,
ice cream, candy, cookies, cake, sodas and breakfast cereals that are high in
sugar. Avoid high-fat cheeses, sour cream, whole milk, butter, mayonnaise,
fried foods and peanut butter (unless it is natural), along with rich salad
dressing. Do not drink alcoholic beverages at all; they are high in calories.

Add healthy fats such as olive oil, safflower oil and flax oil to your diet.
They actually improve fat burning. And drink plenty of water.

Supplements support for weight control
❧   Chromium picolinate: 200–400 mcg
❧   Pyruvate: 6–8 grams per day with diluted fruit juice

- Nature's Secret Ultimate Cleanse: to detoxify
- Whey protein shakes: to help keep blood sugar stable
- Green Tea capsules as a thermogenic
- White willow bark as a thermogenic
- Chickweed as an appetite suppressant
- Horsetail to stimulate the body's metabolism
- Kelp to enhance thyroid function
- Chitosan: a fiber that can bind to fat in the stomach and prevent its absorption (NOTE: Do not take chitosan unless fat is being consumed at a meal.)
- L-carnitine: promotes lean muscle
- L-tyrosine: raises serotonin to inhibit stress or emotional eating
- Ma huang (ephedra) as a thermogenic, very effective. CAUTION: Do not take it late in the day as it may cause insomnia. It is not recommended for those suffering from panic disorder, glaucoma, hypertension or heart disease. And it is safer and more effective to take ma huang when it is combined with other fat burners in a single formula.
- Garcinia Cambogia (Citrin) as an appetite suppressant
- CLA: decreases fat deposition especially in the abdomen. (See Appendix F for valuable information regarding the effectiveness of CLA.)

Lifestyle choices

- Avoid fad diets. They do not work. The results are only temporary.
- Eat slowly and chew your food properly. Take time to taste your food.
- Do not eat when you are upset, lonely or depressed.
- Chewing gum can stimulate your appetite.
- Do not become constipated; use natural remedies to stay regular.
- Begin a walking program (after dinner is best).
- Gradual weight loss is more permanent than quick weight loss. Be patient. The results are more likely to be permanent if the weight loss is a daily gradual process of lifestyle and dietary changes.

WEIGHT LOSS SUCCESS TIPS

- Do not deprive yourself.

- Eat healthy (lots of vegetables, fruits, and whole grains daily).

- An occasional slice of pie will not ruin your progress. Just remember, *occasional* is the key.

- Ask for support.

- Make your friends and family aware of your weight loss goal and enlist their support.

- Turn to friends, family and prayer to help work through any personal problems so that you will not turn to food for comfort.

- Monitor your health. Heed any red flags such as constant fatigue, headache, tension, etc. before they become full-fledged illness.

- Keep up with health screenings, blood pressure, cholesterol screenings, Pap smears, mammograms, dental checkup, skin exams and chiropractic evaluation.

- Find purpose. Fill your life with things that mean more to you than food. Volunteer at church, participate in an outreach program, call your family, your best friend, get involved with passion or cause that you believe in—and dive in!

- Pray. A rich prayer life helps to decrease stress, low self-esteem, social pressures and depression, all of which contribute to overeating.

- Get a diet buddy. If you're trying to change your daily habits without a little help from your friends, you might be missing a very important element. A study in the *Journal of Consulting and Clinical Psychology* found that 95 percent of those who signed up for a weight-loss program with three friends completed the four-month program, compared with 76 percent of those who registered alone. Those who signed up with their friends not only lost more weight than their counterparts, but they also kept it off longer.[76]

ZOONOSIS

Here we are at the end of this family guide, as I promised, with most common ailments, A to Z. Our only Z included here is *zoonosis*. This disease encompasses hundreds of possible diseases that humans contract from animals. Cats, dogs, monkeys, sheep, goats, raccoons, marsupials, elephants, rabbits, pigs and every other thing that was on Noah's ark can potentially infect us with diseases such as anthrax, cowpox, Brucella suis, Q-fever, salmonellosis and more.

Definition
Zoonosis is defined as any disease transmitted from animals to humans.

Symptoms
Symptoms include fever, chills, headaches and flu-like symptoms.

Dietary considerations
Eat a healthy diet of fresh foods, and avoid sugar to keep immunity strong. Drink plenty of water.

Supplement support for zoonosis

- ❦ Vitamin C: 4,000–8,000 mg for one week, then reduce to 3,000 mg daily to fight infection
- ❦ Biotic Silver: a natural antibiotic
- ❦ Kyolic Garlic: a natural antibiotic
- ❦ Vitamin A: 10,000 IU daily
- ❦ Beta carotene: 25,000 IU daily
- ❦ Echinacea tea
- ❦ Goldenseal tea
- ❦ Pau d'arco tea

Lifestyle choices

Seek medical attention if you have been bitten by an animal or if you feel ill after caring for an animal.

Part 4

Self-Tests and Natural Body Maintenance

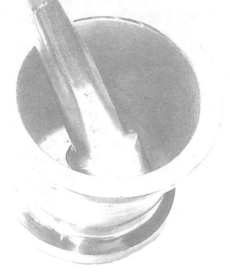

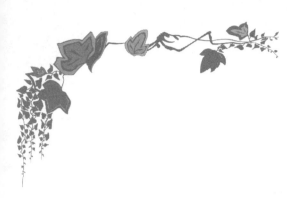

The following section contains self-tests and charts to help you monitor your health or inform you of potential health problems. These tests have been used for many years by natural health professions as a non-invasive way to determine various health conditions that occur in the body. Be sure to work with your healthcare professional if you see that you score high or have several checks on any given test. Again, natural medicine can work hand in hand with conventional medicine. You can use the best of both worlds when it comes to building your health to the highest level possible.

FOR VIBRANT HEALTH PROMISE YOURSELF

To be so strong that nothing can disturb your peace of mind.

To talk health, happiness and prosperity to every person you meet.

To make all your friends feel that there is something in them.

To look at the sunny side of everything and make your optimism come true.

To think only of the best, to work only for the best and expect only the best.

To be just as enthusiastic about the success of others as you are about your own.

To forget the mistakes of the past and press on to the greater achievements of the future.

To wear a cheerful countenance at all times and give every living creature you meet a smile.

To give so much time to improvement of yourself that you have no time to criticize others.

To be too large for worry, too noble for anger, too strong for fear and too happy to permit the presence of trouble.

—AUTHOR UNKNOWN

ADRENAL GLAND FUNCTION TEST

❦ Equipment needed: a home blood pressure monitor.

❦ Lie down and rest for five minutes. Then take your blood pressure while lying still.

❦ Stand up and immediately take another blood pressure reading. If your blood pressure is lower after you stand up, your adrenals are probably functioning poorly. The amount of drop in blood pressure correlates to the amount of adrenal dysfunction.

❦ If you find that your adrenal function is low and that the profile fits you, then take action to nourish and stimulate your adrenal glands. To do so will aid in the healing of hypoglycemia, allergies, exhaustion, fatigue, PMS, menopause, arthritis, bronchitis and will strengthen overall immunity.

STRESS TEST

The following stress test will help you identify stressors in your life and determine the level of stress you may be experiencing at present.[1]

Event		Point Value	Score
1.	Death of spouse	100	_____
2.	Divorce	78	_____
3.	Marital separation	65	_____
4.	Detention in jail	63	_____
5.	Death of close family member other than spouse	63	_____
6.	Major personal injury or illness	53	_____
7.	Marriage	50	_____
8.	Dismissal from job	47	_____
9.	Marital reconciliation	45	_____
10.	Retirement	45	_____
11.	Changes in health or behavior in family member	44	_____
12.	Pregnancy	40	_____
13.	Sexual difficulties	39	_____
14.	Addition to family	39	_____
15.	Major business readjustment	39	_____
16.	Major change in financial status	38	_____
17.	Death of a close friend	37	_____
18.	Change in occupation	36	_____
19.	Change in number of arguments with spouse	35	_____
20.	Going into debt for major purchase	31	_____
21.	Foreclosure of mortgage or loan	30	_____
22.	Major change in responsibility at work	29	_____
23.	Son or daughter leaving home	29	_____
24.	Trouble with in-laws	29	_____
25.	Outstanding personal achievement	28	_____
26.	Spouse begins or ceases work outside the home	26	_____

27.	Beginning or ceasing formal schooling	26	_____
28.	Change in living conditions	25	_____
29.	Revision of personal habits	24	_____
30.	Trouble with your boss	23	_____
31.	Major change in working hours or conditions	20	_____
32.	Change in residence	20	_____
33.	Change in schools	20	_____
34.	Major change in recreational habits	19	_____
35.	Change in religious activities	19	_____
36.	Change in social activities	18	_____
37.	Taking a loan out for smaller purchases	17	_____
38.	Change in sleeping habits	16	_____
39.	Change in number of family gatherings	15	_____
40.	Change in eating habits	15	_____
41.	Vacation	13	_____
42.	Christmas season	12	_____
43.	Minor violation of the law	11	_____
	Total Score		_____

A score below 150 points means statistically that you have a 30 percent chance of developing a significant health problem in the near future. A score between 150 and 300 points gives you a 50 percent chance of developing a significant health problem. A score of more than 300 points raises the possibility of a significant health problem to a whopping 80 percent.

If you scored heavily on the above stress test, you may want to speak with your doctor concerning professional diagnostic tools that are available to measure anxiety levels, such as the Hamilton Anxiety Scale (HAMA). Consult with your physician as well about the possibility of supplementing your diet with a natural aid like GABA, which has been used to calm anxious minds and bodies.

LIVER FLUSH

Since your liver is one of your most important organs, special attention should be given to this hardworking filter of your body. Years ago I was introduced to a very old procedure called the liver and gallbladder flush. This flush improves the immune system by detoxifying the liver and gallbladder. It is a powerful system rejuvenator that helps to restore the liver and gallbladder to normal function.

After personally performing the liver flush on myself, many stones left my body, thereby sparing me pain and discomfort that could have occurred later on. This may seem hard to believe, but the truth is that this procedure has been known for many years and is routinely done by people all over the world.

Many people with gallstones do not realize that they have them. The causes of gallstones are too many fatty and fried foods and the inability to digest them and indigestion from too much dairy, refined sugar, food allergies, high cholesterol sediment, hormone replacement and lack of regular exercise.

The following instructions for the liver and gallbladder flush can be helpful UNLESS your physician has diagnosed you as having large gallstones. This flush is for expelling stones that range in size from a sunflower seed to a cherry pit. Anything larger could be too large to pass through the hepatic duct! So again, this is *not* for large stones. It is a preventative measure that is initially used to expel small stones, and then can be used periodically for maintenance.

- Monday through Saturday noon: Drink as much apple juice as you can in addition to your regular meals and any supplements you are taking. Drink only high-quality apple juice without additives. Purchase a natural juice from the health food store or juice your own organic apples.

- Saturday noon: Eat your normal lunch.

- Three hours later: Take 1 tablespoon of Epsom salt dissolved in ¼ cup of warm water. This acts as a laxative, which will help the expulsion process. Now, I must warn you, Epsom salt does not taste very good, so drink a little fresh grapefruit juice right after.

- Two hours later: Repeat, with 1 teaspoon of Epsom salt dissolved in ¼ cup warm water, followed by fresh grapefruit juice.

- Dinner Saturday night: Have grapefruit juice for your meal.

- Bedtime: Drink ½ cup of warm unrefined olive oil. I prefer extra-virgin olive oil. Blend this with ½ cup of fresh lemon juice.

- After this, go directly to bed. Lie on your right side with your knees pulled up close to your chest for thirty minutes. Keep in mind that it is perfectly normal to experience nausea after drinking this olive oil mixture. It will pass as you fall asleep.

   ✻   Sunday morning: One hour before breakfast, take 1 tablespoon of Epsom salt dissolved in ¼ cup warm water. After this you may go back to your regular, healthy eating plan.

   ✻   When you have your next bowel movement, you should notice small gallstone-type objects in the stool. They range in color from light to dark green and in size from sunflower seeds to cherry pits. Most people find this absolutely amazing. Most skeptics become real proponents of the flush.

   ✻   If you see a large number of stones, the flush should be repeated in about one month.

I recommend the liver flush once a year for maintenance. This flush is a very important self-treatment. When your liver is clean and functioning well, the whole body benefits. This procedure falls under the category of something that you have to see to believe.

BOWEL FUNCTION TEST

Occasionally, after a detoxification program, some people experience bowel sluggishness. It is imperative that you continue to have at least two to three bowel movements per day to keep the cleansing and regeneration process moving forward smoothly. How do you accomplish this? The answer is easy enough. Just make sure that you are getting enough fiber in your diet. A good indicator of adequate fiber intake is as follows:[2]

   ✻   Bowel movement two to three times daily
   ✻   Stool should float
   ✻   Stool should be almost odorless
   ✻   Bowel movement should be effortless, no straining
   ✻   No flatulence

Keep in mind that when you eventually eat more fiber or take a fiber supplement, you may initially experience flatulence as your body adjusts. Please make sure to drink plenty of water as usual. This is especially true when you increase your fiber intake. By making sure that your fiber intake is what it should be, you are helping to prevent dreaded ailments, such as bowel cancer, colitis, constipation, diverticulitis and hemorrhoids. Just remember the stool criteria. If you see that you are offtrack, simply add more fiber supplements until your bowel movements are what they should be.

FOODS HIGH IN FIBER

Oatmeal	Plum	Almonds
Corn—cooked	Apple with skin	Carrots—cooked
Brown rice	Pinto beans	Nectarine
Dates	Banana	Brazil nuts
Raw pineapple	Raisins	Cooked spinach
Papaya	Blueberries	Honeydew
Whole cranberries	Lima beans	Bran
Dried prunes	Seeds and nuts	Raw vegetables
Whole-grain cereals	Potato with skin	Brussels sprouts
	—baked	—cooked

Commercial fiber supplements:
Nature's Secret Ultimate Fiber Powder

EAR CANDLING—AN ANCIENT TECHNIQUE

Imagine, if you can, a hollow candle that can get rid of inches of impacted earwax, candida infections and fungus. Imagine a candle that could be an alternative to surgery. Imagine a candle that has the power to improve and return hearing, improve physical balance, cleanse the sinus cavities and the lymphatic system, cleanse toxins left by medications, eliminate ear pains and promote healthier ears.

An ancient technique exists called ear candling, which is still practiced effectively today. And it's sweeping the country like wildfire. All over America, people can't seem to get enough of it. The technique is so easy that all it requires are two candles and a little common sense.

What is ear candling?

Ear candling is an ancient technique that has been around for thousands of years. Many think it is started with the ancient Egyptians, who searched for reeds in the Nile River so they could clean and dry out their ears. Because of the success of this technique, it quickly spread to other parts of the globe, such as China, Greece and even South America. Now, it is commonly practiced in many places.

In fact, here in the United States, ear candling was a popular American folk remedy. The participants wrapped newspapers around gun cleaning rods, dipped them in wax or glue and next removed the rod. What they had left was a hollow tube of wax used as an ear candle. In Germany, candling is taught as a valid ear-cleaning procedure to medical students. Ear candling stands in a class of its own when it comes to natural healing.

This truly amazing technique utilizes a hollow candle coated with wax. The instructions are simple. One end of the candle is placed snugly into the ear, and the other end is the one you light. The lighting of the candle creates a gentle vacuum that can soften and dislodge wax and debris and pull it into the candle.

The principle of this procedure is very simple. When the candle is placed in the ear canal and lit, the flame warms the air inside the cylinder and produces a vacuum. Obviously, the flame needs oxygen, and in order to feed it oxygen, the air inside the candle must rise upward. This in turn creates suction and airflow through the ear canal.

Ear candling is a very effective way you can totally cleanse your ears. There is debris inside the ears that cannot be reached with fingertips or Q-tips alone. Impacted wax, fungus, past residues of infection, fat globules and more build up in the ear and hide in the crevices. For example, people who have candida yeast typically have an accumulation of fungus in the ears. Because the ear is dark and moist, it provides a perfect environment for yeast to breed. It is close to the blood supply that comes up into the head and therefore is supplied by a major food source.

Candling is not limited to sick persons or those afflicted by ear problems. Just like regular body maintenance, such as clipping the fingernails, brushing the teeth or combing the hair, everyone can benefit from having their ears cleaned. Most people do not truly realize exactly how much "gunk" is in the ears until they undergo their first ear-candling session. You will be very surprised at the amount of stuff that has been hiding in the grooves of the ears since the time of birth. It gets into the hard-to-reach areas where the fungus and wax has become impacted and hardened.

How often should the ears be cleaned? The length of time between each ear candling session depends upon the condition of the ears. For general cleaning purposes, simply to keep the ears in good healthy shape, once every couple of months will do just fine. If the problem is more severe, such as difficulty hearing, three sessions can be done three to seven days apart from one another. This allows the ear time to replenish its normal wax and, in addition, stimulate its own healing naturally.

CAUTION: Never do ear candling alone; always have someone with you.

Candida Test

To see if candida overgrowth could be contributing to your current state of health, take the following yeast screening developed by William Crook, M.D.

Yeast Screening

Section A: History

For *yes* answers apply the points in the parenthesis. *No* answers equal zero points.

1. Have you taken Tetracycline or other antibiotics for acne one month or longer? (35 points) _____
2. Have you at any time in your life taken broad-spectrum antibiotics or other antibacterial medication for respiratory, urinary or other infections for two months of longer, or in shorter courses, four or more times in a one-year period? (35 points) _____
3. Have you taken a broad-spectrum antibiotic drug even in a single dose? (6 points) _____
4. Have you at any time in your life been bothered by persistent prostatitis, vaginitis or other problems affecting your reproductive organs? (25 points) _____
5. Are you bothered by memory or concentration problems? Do you sometimes feel spaced out? (20 points) _____
6. Do you feel "sick all over," yet in spite of visits to many physicians, the causes haven't been found? (20 points) _____
7. Have you been pregnant two or more times? (5 points) _____
   One time? (3 points) _____
8. Have you taken birth control pills…
   For more than two years? (15 points) _____
   For six months to two years? (8 points) _____
9. Have you taken steroids orally, by injection or inhalation?
   For more than two weeks? (15 points) _____
   For two weeks or less? (6 points) _____
10. Does exposure to perfumes, insecticides, fabric shop odors and other chemicals provoke moderate to severe symptoms? (20 points) _____
    Mild symptoms?(5 points) _____
11. Does tobacco smoke really bother you? (10 points) _____
12. Are your symptoms worse on damp, muggy days or in moldy places? (20 points) _____
13. Have you had athlete's foot, ringworm, "jock itch" or other chronic fungus infections of the skin or nails? (10 points) _____
    Have such infections been severe or persistent? (20 points) _____
    Mild to moderate? (10 points) _____
14. Do you crave sugar? (10 points) _____
    Total Score Section A _____

SECTION B: MAJOR SYMPTOMS

These symptoms are often present in persons with yeast-connected health challenges.

    Scoring system for section B:
Occasional or mild = 3 points
Frequent and/or moderately severe = 6 points
Severe and/or disabling = 9 points

1. Fatigue or lethargy   _____
2. Feeling of being "drained"   _____
3. Depression or manic depression   _____
4. Numbness, burning or tingling   _____
5. Headaches   _____
6. Muscle aches   _____
7. Muscle weakness or paralysis   _____
8. Pain and/or swelling in joints   _____
9. Abdominal pain   _____
10. Bloating, belching or intestinal gas   _____
11. Constipation and/or diarrhea   _____
12. Troublesome vaginal burning, itching or discharge   _____
13. Prostatitis   _____
14. Impotence   _____
15. Loss of sexual desire or feeling   _____
16. Endometriosis   _____
17. Cramps and/or other menstrual irregularities   _____
18. Premenstrual tension   _____
19. Attacks of anxiety or crying   _____
20. Cold hands or feet, low body temperature   _____
21. Hypothyroidism   _____
22. Shaking or irritable when hungry   _____
23. Cystitis or interstitial cystitis   _____
    Total Score Section B   _____

SECTION C

These are additional yeast-related symptoms.

    Scoring system for Section C:
Occasional or mild = 1 point
Frequent or moderately severe = 2 points
Severe and/or disabling = 3 points

1. Drowsiness, including inappropriate drowsiness   _____
2. Irritability   _____
3. Uncoordination   _____
4. Frequent mood swings   _____
5. Insomnia   _____
6. Dizziness or loss of balance   _____
7. Pressure above ears/feeling of head swelling   _____
8. Sinus problems/tenderness of cheekbones or forehead   _____
9. Tendency to bruise easily   _____

10. Eczema, itching eyes   _____
11. Psoriasis   _____
12. Chronic hives   _____
13. Indigestion or heartburn   _____
14. Sensitivity to milk, wheat, corn or other common foods   _____
15. Mucus in stools   _____
16. Rectal itching   _____
17. Dry mouth or throat   _____
18. Mouth rashes, including "white tongue"   _____
19. Bad breath   _____
20. Foot, hair or body odor not relieved by washing   _____
21. Nasal congestion or postnasal drip   _____
22. Nasal itching   _____
23. Sore throat   _____
24. Laryngitis or loss of voice   _____
25. Cough or recurrent bronchitis   _____
26. Pain or tightness in chest   _____
27. Wheezing or shortness of breath   _____
28. Urinary frequency or urgency   _____
29. Burning on urination   _____
30. Spots in front of eyes or erratic vision   _____
31. Burning or tearing eyes   _____
32. Recurrent infections or fluid in ears   _____
33. Ear pain or deafness   _____
     Total Score Section C   _____

     Total Score: Section A   _____
                  Section B   _____
                  Section C   _____
     GRAND TOTAL SCORE   _____

How did you score?

Women with a score over 180 and men with a score over 140 almost certainly have yeast-connected health problems. Women with a score over 120 and men with a score over 90 *probably* have yeast-connected health problems. Women with a score over 60 and men with a score over 40 possibly have yeast-connected health problems. Women with a score less than 60 and men with a score less than 40 are less apt to have yeast-connected health problems.

Most of the people that I have worked with in my office have scored very high on the yeast questionnaire. Most of these people are the product of the "antibiotic era."

Enzyme Test

Use the following to determine which enzymes you need to start adding to your program.

Amylase deficiency

- ❏ Breaking out of the skin, rash
- ❏ Hypoglycemia
- ❏ Depression
- ❏ Mood swings
- ❏ Allergies
- ❏ Inflammation
- ❏ PMS
- ❏ Hot flashes
- ❏ Fatigue
- ❏ Cold hands and feet
- ❏ Neck and shoulder aches
- ❏ Sprue

Protease deficiency

- ❏ Back weakness
- ❏ Fungal forms
- ❏ Constipation
- ❏ High blood pressure
- ❏ Insomnia
- ❏ Hearing problems
- ❏ Parasites
- ❏ Gum disorders
- ❏ Gingivitis

Lipase deficiency

- ❏ Aching feet
- ❏ Arthritis
- ❏ Bladder problems
- ❏ Cystitis
- ❏ Acne
- ❏ Gallbladder stress
- ❏ Gallstones
- ❏ Hay fever
- ❏ Prostate problems
- ❏ Psoriasis
- ❏ Urinary weakness
- ❏ Constipation
- ❏ Diarrhea
- ❏ Heart problems

Combination deficiency

- ❏ Chronic allergies
- ❏ Common colds
- ❏ Immune depressed conditions
- ❏ Irritable bowel
- ❏ Chronic fatigue
- ❏ Sinus infection
- ❏ Diverticulitis

Once you determine your particular enzyme deficiency, you may then choose the Enzymedica plant enzyme formula that best suits your profile.

STRESS RELIEF

I have found in my own life, when faced with stress and tension, that my muscles tighten all over my body and I generally feel miserable. I began research into muscle tension and found that physical and emotional stress gets stored in your muscles, making you more tense. Fortunately, there are natural solutions when you feel yourself tightening up.

Massage therapy has a long history of therapeutic benefits. A stressed body responds beautifully to regular massage therapy sessions. If this sounds a bit impractical for you, do not worry; there is always exercise, like walking, stretching and light weightlifting. But I want to share with you a wonderful technique that will work for you time and time again when you are faced with a body that is tight with stressed muscles.

Your "MANTLE" for stress relief

I call it the "MANTLE Technique," and I am using it even as I am writing this book to relieve the tightness in my neck and shoulders. What is it? It is very simple. My "MANTLE Technique" is simply tensing and holding for the count of ten each part of your body one section at a time. To remind myself that I need attention daily, I created the acronym MANTLE.

M - muscles
A - always
N - need
T – tension
L - loosening
E – every day

So, begin with your eyes. Close your eyes; tense and hold for ten seconds, then release. Take a deep cleansing breath. Try to belly breathe. Fill your diaphragm with air and exhale slowly through your mouth.

Next, tighten all of the muscles of your face and mouth; make a face, and hold it for ten seconds. Take another cleansing deep breath. Continue this tensing and releasing exercise on down to the other parts of your body, including neck, shoulders, arms, hands, fingers, stomach, lower abdomen, upper thighs, calves, feet and toes. After each area has been relaxed, take time for prayer and reflection as well.

Quick relaxer: self-massage

To ease your neck muscles, place your thumbs at the base of your skull, just below your ears. Press inward and upward for six seconds, then release. Repeat, moving your thumbs a quarter inch inward along the base of your skull each time.

To reach your lower back, put four tennis balls in a sock. Place the sock at the base of your back, lie down and roll gently for a few minutes. Your body weight applies the pressure.

To relax your shoulders, place your fingertips on your shoulders at the base of your neck. Press down; hold the pressure for six seconds. Release, then repeat, gradually working your fingers down your shoulder line.

Body work: stress-relieving baths

If you are suffering from too little sleep, high stress levels, poor diet, too much caffeine or alcohol, or frequent flu or colds, this bath will alkalinize an over-acid body. Refer to pages 25 and 64 for therapeutic baths, and follow instructions for the salt and soda bath. You will feel remarkably energized and refreshed. This should be taken periodically to keep your acid-alkaline level in balance. Pain and stress cause acidity in the body, which can translate into degenerative disease. This bath can help prevent needless suffering.

Appendix A

Ten Popular Homeopathic Remedies

1. *Aconite,* derived from the monkshood plant, is used for anxiety and colds. For colds, take one dose four times daily for two to three days; for best results, take it at the first sign of your symptoms. For anxiety, take one dose four times daily. If anxiety persists beyond one week, refer to the anxiety section on page 105.

2. *Arnica,* derived from the mountain daisy, is used for swelling, bruising from a fall or blow, or for pain. Take one dose an hour for three hours, starting immediately or as soon as possible after an injury, then twice daily until bruising, swelling and pain subside. It is excellent for sports injuries like sprains, strains and stiffness.

3. *Arsenicum album,* derived from white arsenic (a mineral) is used for colds, minor infections, vomiting or diarrhea, and ailments characterized by restlessness and/or burning pain. For colds, take one dose four times daily for two to three days. For diarrhea or vomiting, take one dose after each episode.

4. *Belladonna* is used for headache, menstrual cramps, children's fever or earache. For headache or menstrual cramps, take one dose every one to two hours for up to three doses. For fever or earache, take one dose every two to three hours.

5. *Bryonia,* derived from wild hops, is used for minor injuries, coughing or influenza. For an injury, take one dose every two to three hours for two to three days until healing is complete. For flu, take one dose six times a day for two days. For cough, take one dose four times daily for two to three days.

6. *Hepar sulfur,* derived from calcium salts, is used for sinus infections, sore throat and sharp throat pain with chills. For a sore throat, take one dose every two to three hours for up to twenty-four hours. For sinus infections, take one dose every two to three hours for relief within eight hours.

7. *Ignatia* is primarily a female remedy to relax and relieve emotional tension. It is especially helpful during grief or loss. For tension, take one dose every hour for up to three doses until tension is alleviated. For grief, take one dose every hour up to three doses as needed.

8. *Nux vomica,* derived from the poison nut plant, is good for indigestion, colds, light and noise sensitivity, flatulence, constipation and motion sickness. For indigestion, take one dose every one to two hours for up to three doses. For colds, take one dose four times daily for two to three days.

9. *Pulsatilla,* derived from the wind flower plant, is good for weepy or clingy children, colds, children's fever, earache or pink eye. For earache, pink eye or fever, take one dose every two to three hours. NOTE: If no improvement occurs after three doses or if pain persists, see your doctor.

10. *Rhus tox,* derived from poison ivy, is good for chicken pox, swollen, stiff joints, strains and sprains, hives, burns and rashes. It also helps alleviate poison ivy. For chicken pox, take one dose four to six times daily. If no improvement occurs, then try pulsatilla.

HOW TO TAKE A HOMEOPATHIC REMEDY

❧ All homeopathic remedies should be stored at room temperature away from heat, sunlight, perfumes, camphor, plants and liniments as these things will weaken the remedies' effectiveness.

❧ Repeat the remedy as needed. You may experience a mild "healing crisis" or aggravation of symptoms initially when you repeat the dose. Do not be alarmed; this will pass.

❧ Do not eat or drink anything ten minutes after taking a remedy. Homeopathic remedies enter the bloodstream through your mouth's mucous membranes. The remedies are usually in liquid or tablet form. For best results, take ½ dropperful under the tongue and hold for thirty seconds before you swallow. Allow tablets to dissolve under the tongue.

❧ Homeopathic remedies are available in a variety of strengths or dilutions. More is not necessarily better when it comes to homeopathic remedies. Smaller doses over a period of time are more effective. They should be discontinued when healing has occurred.

APPENDIX B

------◆·▪·◆------

AMINO AMMO

The following amino acids also help to restore and replenish the brain.

* *Lysine* is effective in the natural treatment of hypothyroidism, Alzheimer's disease and Parkinson's disease.

* *Glutamine* is a prime brain nutrient and energy source. Supplementing your brain with glutamine can rapidly improve memory, recall, concentration and alertness. It helps to reduce sugar and alcohol cravings and controls hypoglycemic reactions.

* *GABA* stores must be replaced on a regular basis since anxiety, pain and grief are a daily occurrence and deplete the GABA reserves; it must be replenished each day. GABA improves brain function and reduces anxiety.

* *Tyrosine* is a wonderful semi-essential amino acid formed from phenylalanine. Tyrosine helps to build the body's natural supply of adrenaline and thyroid hormones. It is also an antioxidant and a source of quick energy, especially for the brain. Because it converts in the body to the amino acid L-dopa, it is considered a safe natural support for Parkinson's disease, depression and hypertension. NOTE: If you have cancerous melanoma or suffer from manic depression, you should avoid tyrosine.

* *Glycine* helps to release growth hormone when taken in large doses. It converts to creatine in the body to retard nerve and muscle degeneration. It is wonderful for controlling and regulating hypoglycemic sugar drops, especially effective when taken in the morning upon rising.

* *Taurine*, a potent anti-seizure amino acid, is a neurotransmitter that helps control the nervous system and hyperactivity, normalizes irregular heartbeat, helps prevent circulatory and heart disorders and helps to lower cholesterol. Since the natural sources of taurine are hard to find, supplementation is the best way to receive adequate amounts for therapeutic benefit.

Guidelines for Taking Amino Acids

❦   Take amino acids with their nutrient cofactors for the best uptake.

❦   Take amino acids before meals, with the exception of brain stimulant amino acids.

❦   Make sure to take amino acids with plenty of water for optimum absorption.

❦   Please note that active forms of amino acids are only available for sale, so even if you do not see an "L- (levo) or D- (dextro)" before the amino acid, the product is still the active form. Example: L-carnitine or carnitine.

APPENDIX C

STRESS BUSTERS FROM NATURE

SIBERIAN GINSENG

Siberian ginseng is a root that belongs to the ginseng family of adaptogenic herbs. Adaptogens help build our resistance to stress. Siberian ginseng helps the body adapt to stress and lessens fatigue, often two underlying factors in the anxiety picture. It improves oxygen and blood sugar metabolism as well as immune function. The recommended dosage is 180 to 360 milligrams of Siberian ginseng extract standardized to 0.8 percent eleutherosides, in two equally divided doses. Take daily for two to three months, then take a two-week break before resuming.

Since Siberian ginseng is a stimulant, do not take it before bed or if you have high blood pressure. It is not helpful for severe anxiety. See your doctor if your symptoms are severe. One last tip: Do not confuse Siberian ginseng with Panax ginseng, because Panax ginseng can increase your levels of cortisol (the body's stress hormone).

VALERIAN

Valerian is widely used in Europe as a sedative. It is also used to treat nervous conditions and insomnia in Chinese medicine. Its effect is said to be similar to benzodiazepine tranquilizers, but without side effects. Valerian works like benzodiazepines by enhancing the activity of GABA, the naturally tranquilizing neurotransmitter. The dosage is 300 to 900 milligrams of valerian extract (standardized to 0.8 percent valeric acid) taken one hour before bedtime for insomnia.

Taking 50 to 100 milligrams two to three times a day may help relieve performance anxiety and stress. Do not take valerian with alcohol. Side effects are rare, but they may include headache and stimulant effects in some people. The effects of valerian use are cumulative, so you have to take it for two to three weeks before evaluating your results. I call valerian "God's sleeping pill."

PASSIONFLOWER

Passionflower is a climbing plant, native to North America. Passionflower combined with valerian is a popular herbal remedy throughout much of Europe for insomnia, anxiety and irritability.

ST. JOHN'S WORT

St. John's wort has been used to treat anxiety and depression in Europe for more than twenty-four hundred years. Pretty impressive, wouldn't you say? Once again here is a natural substance that enhances the activity of GABA. In addition, St. John's wort enhances the activity of three important neurotransmitters: serotonin, norepinephrine and dopamine.

In a study published in the *British Medical Journal* in 1996, St. John's wort proved to be an effective treatment for mild to moderately severe depression with almost zero side effects.[1] The standardized dose is 300 milligrams extract (standardized to 0.3 percent hypericin) three times per day. St. John's wort must be taken for six weeks before evaluating your results because the effect is cumulative and not immediate.

NOTE: Do not take St. John's wort if you are currently taking prescription antidepressants, especially MAO inhibitors (Nardil, Parnate). If you are taking a prescription antidepressant, check with your healthcare practitioner before stopping the medication. If you stop taking a prescription antidepressant, wait at least four weeks before taking St. John's wort to make sure that no overlapping occurs. Side effects are very rare, but include dizziness and gastrointestinal irritation.

KAVA

The root of Piper Methysticum, this member of the pepper tree is native to the South Pacific area. Kava proved superior to placebo for both short-term and long-term treatment. Anxiety, tension, fear and insomnia decreased steadily during the course of treatment according to a 1997 randomized placebo-controlled, multi-center study published in *Pharmacopsychiatry* where outpatients took 70 milligrams of kavalactones or a placebo.[2]

Kava has a natural tranquilizing effect on the brain by producing a soothing effect in the amygdala, the "alarm center" of the brain. The recommended dosage is 70 to 85 milligrams (70 percent kavalactones), taken in the evening. You may increase the dose to as much as 100 milligrams three times daily if necessary.

Do not mix kava with alcohol, pharmaceutical antidepressants, benzodiazepine, tranquilizers or sleeping pills. If you have Parkinson's disease, you should not take kava because it may worsen muscular weakness. Extremely high doses of kava (ten times the normal dose) can cause problems with vision, breathing and muscles. Yellowing and scaly skin has also occurred at high doses. Kava, if used properly, can bring blessed relief.[3]

5-HTP

5-HTP, derived from the seed of the *Griffonia* tree and related to the amino acid tryptophan, is used to treat anxiety, insomnia, depression and other related conditions linked with low levels of serotonin. 5-HTP is a raw material the body uses to manufacture serotonin, the neurotransmitter linked with mood. By raising serotonin levels in the body, anxiety and depression can be relieved. Informal studies suggest that 5-HTP is effective for mild to moderate anxiety as well as for full-blown anxiety disorders.

The most effective study dose range was 75–100 milligrams per day. You should start with 25 milligrams per day at the time of the day when you feel most anxious. If you are interested in learning more about 5-HTP, I highly recommend the book *5-HTP: Nature's Serotonin Solution.*[4]

WHICH WAY TO GO: DRUGS OR HERBS?

Ultimately, you have to decide to treat your body naturally or to use prescription drugs. Talk to your physician before discontinuing any prescription medication. The following chart serves as a general guideline of natural alternatives to prescribed drugs.

GUIDELINES FOR NATURAL ALTERNATIVES TO DRUGS

FOR MODERATE TO SEVERE ANXIETY AND CHRONIC STRESS

Prescription Drugs	Herbal Alternatives
Xanax	Kava
Valium	Valerian
Klonopin	Siberian ginseng as an adaptogen
Ativan	Passionflower
Tranxene	L-Theanine
Sleeping pills (Restoril, Dalmane, Halcion, Serax)	

FOR DEPRESSION AND ANXIETY

Prescription Drugs	Herbal Alternatives
SSRIs—Paxil	St. John's wort
Prozac	5-HTP
Zoloft	

In most cases, costs of prescription drugs are much higher than the cost of using natural herbal remedies. And natural herbs do not cause the side effects of weight gain, sexual dysfunction, insomnia, nausea, nervousness, agitation, sweating or heart palpitation that sometimes accompany prescription drugs.

NATURAL PROTOCOL FOR STRESS

T he following natural substances along with their dosages are recommended to help combat the effects of stress.

GABA

Since the amino acid GABA affects our mind, memory, mood and behavior, along with the fact that stress, trauma and anxiety deplete our supply of GABA, I recommend that you supplement with GABA. GABA has a natural calming effect and helps to cool the brain. Remember that amino acid deficiencies occur when we experience long periods of pain, stress, depression or anxiety. Once depletion occurs, the brain is then overwhelmed by anxiety signals, leaving you tense and out of control.

Your brain needs more than 100 milligrams daily of GABA to restore it to the proper level. I recommend capsules over tablets for easier assimilation. (This is true for all of my supplement recommendations.)

LIQUID SEROTONIN

If you are not currently on SSRI medication, commonly known as selective serotonin reuptake inhibitors, you may take liquid serotonin. Serotonin is a key neurotransmitter in brain function that enhances focus, elevates mood, reduces anger and aggression, and can help reduce cravings for carbohydrates and alcohol.

L-THEANINE

Take 100–400 milligrams to induce a state of relaxation.

MAGNESIUM GEL CAPS

Take 400 milligrams at bedtime. Low magnesium levels are found in persons with hyperirritability, depression and anxiety. In addition, magnesium helps to relax the muscles.

BRAIN LINK

Brain Link is a total amino acid complex that blankets your system with all of the amino acids that create neurotransmitter links for enhanced brain function. Used daily, it is a total formula that can be used along with the abovementioned supplements.

ANXIETY CONTROL 24

This is an amino acid support formula that contains amino acids, herbs, vitamins and minerals, along with essential cofactors to help relax the anxious mind or stressed body. Billie J. Sahley formulated the formula. It contains the herbs passionflower and *Primula officinalis,* which support an overstressed body and calm the central nervous system naturally. It is a formula that can be used day or night to fill the deficiencies caused by our stressful lives. It is also wonderful for anxious or active teens. I only wish I had this formula during my teen years!

VITAMIN B$_6$

Vitamin B$_6$ must be taken with all amino acids. You may take a B-complex formula, which contains vitamin B$_6$ along with the full spectrum of B vitamins.

APPENDIX E

TIPS FOR
BEATING STRESS

Do you feel a need to work on your stress level? Try these suggestions:

- *Simplify your life.* Take inventory of how you spend your time, money and energy, and determine whether you really want or need everything you currently invest in. Can anything go without sacrificing personal or family happiness? Cut unnecessary stressful activities out of your life. Say *no* the next time you are asked to take on a new responsibility if you are already overextended from doing too much.

- *Get enough sleep.* Most people don't. If you have trouble falling asleep, an evening routine can help you. Don't drink caffeine or exercise late in the day, and keep a regular bedtime, adjusting it no more than an hour on weekends.

- *Eat well.* Besides choosing healthy foods, make mealtimes a pleasant social encounter. Celebrate family time by making menu planning, table setting and cooking together family activities.

- *Exercise.* It triggers chemical reactions in our bodies, it enhances our moods, it makes us more fit to handle physical challenges, and it doesn't have to be structured. Look for opportunities to move—park farther from your destination for a longer walk, take the stairs instead of the elevator, toss a ball with your family in the backyard.

- *Have fun.* Keep good a balance of work and play and of solitary and group activities. Sometimes we need time alone to gather our thoughts; sometimes we need people around to hug, listen to or share ideas with us.

- *Maintain a support system.* Make sure your schedule accommodates time with loved ones. Think of recreational activities you can do with friends or family that don't cost much. If you struggle with a disease or circumstance such as single parenthood, join a support group.

❦ *Meditate and pray.* Find ways to focus energy on a meaning and purpose beyond your everyday life.

❦ *Keep your sense of humor.* Laughter releases tension. Look for what's funny in everyday life. Find classic comedies on television or the library's video section.

❦ *Be assertive.* Don't bottle up negative emotions and experiences. When you have a difficult message to deliver, describe the situation, express your feelings, specify your wants and say it directly to the person involved. Write it down first or practice verbally if that will help.

❦ *Be creative.* Indulge in enjoyable hobbies, whether they be painting, gardening, dancing, writing in a journal or singing in a church choir or by yourself.

❦ *Give of yourself.* Finding a way to help someone in need is the best way to remind ourselves to be grateful for what we might take for granted.

❦ *Pamper yourself.* It doesn't cost much to relax with a long bubble bath, a foot bath while reading the mail or a series of family back rubs.

CLA = Weight Loss

Conjugated linoleic acid (CLA) used to be found in abundant amounts in red meat, butter and cheese. Today, there is less CLA in dairy products because most cows are artificially fattened in feedlots instead of grazing on grass. Many Americans also consume less red meat, butter and dairy foods. The result is that people are obtaining only a fraction of CLA compared to previous generations.

CLA has shown strong anticancer properties, being particularly effective in inhibiting breast and prostate tumors, as well as colorectal, stomach and skin cancer, including melanoma. What makes CLA unique is that even low concentrations inhibit growth of cancer cells.

CLA supplementation has been shown to improve the lean mass to body fat ratio, decreasing fat deposition, especially in the abdomen, and enhancing muscle growth. One mechanism by which CLA reduces body fat is to prevent the excess accumulation of glucose and fatty acids in the body's adipocytes (fat cells). People become fatter when the volume of their adipocytes expands. CLA also facilitates fat loss by improving insulin sensitivity and increasing energy expenditure.

The amount of CLA used in human weight-loss studies was 3,000 milligrams of pure CLA. Therefore, you will need to take at least 3,000–4,000 milligrams daily, but be sure to take it all at once and early in the day.

Health Update — Rev Up Fat-Burning Potential

Conjugated linoleic acid (CLA) reduces body fat by increasing your basal metabolic rate. In the August 2001 *Journal of Obesity,* a study of twenty-five men showed that CLA is effective in reducing abdominal fat.[1] Carnitine and chromium increase the rate in which fat is burned. These three supplements effectively support body weight management.

NOTES

CHAPTER 1: NATURAL MEDICINE 101

1. Robert C. Atkins, M.D., *Dr. Atkins' New Diet Revolution* (New York: M. Evans and Company, Inc., 1999), 76.
2. James F. Balch, M.D. and Phyllis Balch, *Prescription for Nutritional Healing* (Garden City, NY: Avery Publishing Group, 1997), 6.

CHAPTER 3: YOUR TOOLBOX FOR BUILDING HEALTH

1. The Burton Goldberg Group, *Alternative Medicine: The Definitive Guide* (Puyallup, WA: Future Medicine Publishing, 1994), 157.
2. Linda Page, *Healthy Healing*, 11th ed. (n.p.: Traditional Wisdom, Inc., 2000), 170.
3. National Diabetes Statistics: General Information and National Estimates on Diabetes in the United States, 2000, NIH Publication No. 02-3892 (March 2002).
4. "Stevia: An (Illegal) Sweetener," *Reach for Life Journal* (March/April 1997).
5. Ibid.
6. Paul Stamets, *Growing Gourmet and Medicinal Mushrooms* (n.p.: Ten Speed Publishing, 1994).
7. Christopher Hobbs, *Medicinal Mushrooms* (Santa Cruz, CA: Botanical Press, 1995).
8. *Energy Times* (November/December 1999); *The Townsend Letter* (June 1998); Stamets, *Growing Gourmet and Medicinal Mushrooms*.
9. James Balch, M.D. and Phyllis Balch, *Rx For Cooking and Dietary Wellness* (n.p.: PAB Books, Inc., 1992).
10. A. Casey et al., "Creatine ingestion favorably affects performance and muscle metabolism during maximal exercise in humans," *Am. J. Physiol.* 271 (July 1996): E31–E37.
11. Y. Park et al., "Effect of conjugated linoleic acid on body composition in mice," *Lipids* 32 (August 1997): 853–858.
12. J. F. Flood et al., "Pregnenolone sulfate enhances past training memory when injected in very low doses into limbic system structures; the amygdala is by far the most sensitive," *Proc. Natl. Acad. Sci., USA* 92 (November 7, 1995): 10806–10810.
13. K. Zmilacher et al., "L–5-Hydroxytryptophan alone and in combination with a peripheral decarboxylase inhibitor in the treatment of depression," *Neuropsychobiology* 20 (1988): 28–35.
14. C. R. Pace-Asciak et al., "The red wine phenolics transresveratrol and quercetin block human platelet aggregation and elcosanoid synthesis: implications for protection against coronary heart disease," *Clin. Chim. Acta.* 235 (March 31, 1995): 207–219.
15. O. Kanauhi et al., "Mechanism for the inhibition of fat digestion by chitosan and for the synergistic effect of ascorbate," *Biosci. Biotechrol. Biochem* 59 (May 1995): 786–790.
16. H. Langsjoen et al., "Usefulness of Coenzyme Q10 in clinical cardiology: a long-term study," *Mol. Aspects Med.* 15 Suppl (1994): S165–S175.
17. H. P. Fleming et al., "Antimicrobial properties of oleuropein and products of its hydrolysis from green olives," *Appl. Microbiol.* 26 (November 1973): 777–782.
18. M. E. Attenburrow et al., "Low dose melatonin improves sleep in middle-aged subjects," *Psychopharmacology* 126 (July 1996): 179–181.
19. Cenacchi et al., "Cognitive decline in the elderly; a double-blind, placebo-controlled multicenter study on efficacy of phosphatidylserine administration," *Aging* (Milano) 5 (April 1993): 123–133.
20. Balch and Balch, *Prescription for Nutritional Healing*.

21.   DicQie Fuller, Ph.D., D.Sc., *The Healing Power of Enzymes* (New York: Forbes Custom Publishing, 1998), 10.

Chapter 4: Natural Healing Protocols

1.   Retrieved from the Internet, 9/20/02: www.nelsonbach.com/bachessences/pages/frame01.htm

Part 2: Determine Your Personal Health Needs

1.   Sylvia Kreutle, M.S. *Nutritional Symptomatology Questionnaire*. Fort Collins, CO: HealthQuest, Inc. Used by permission. (For more information, see www.hquest.com.)

Part 3: Family Health Remedies: A-to-Z Guide

1.   "Rabbi Ben Ezra" by Robert Browning.
2.   Robert M. Giller, M.D. and Kathy Matthews, *Medical Makeover* (New York: William Morrow and Company, 1989), 236–252.
3.   *The World's Greatest Treasury of Health Secrets*, ed. Boardline, Inc. (Greenwich, CT: Bottomline Books, 2002), 272.
4.   Source retrieved from the Internet October 22, 2002: "Herbs Can Spice Up Your Antioxidant Protection," *LifeExtension Daily News* (April 18, 2002): www.leforg/newsarchive/nutrition.
5.   Source retrieved from the Internet October 22, 2002: "Researchers Report Vitamin # Protects Key Proteins From Damage Due to Aging," Arizona Health Sciences Center, University of Arizona (May 28, 1996): www.ahsc.arizona.edu/opa/news/may96/kay.htm.
6.   Balch and Balch, *Prescription for Nutritional Healing*, 123.
7.   Mary Sano et al., "A Controlled Trial of Selegiline, Alpha-Tocopherol, or Both as Treatment for Alzheimer's Disease," *New England Journal of Medicine* 336 (April 24, 1997): 1216–1222. Retrieved from the Internet October 11, 2002 at www.content.nejm.org.
8.   Source retrieved from the Internet October 22, 2002: "Estrogen May Delay Alzheimer's Onset in Postmenopausal Women," *Columbia University Record* 22 (September 13, 1996): www.columbia.edu/cu/1996/0913/d.html.
9.   Source retried from the Internet October 22, 2002: "Anti-inflammatories reduce risks of Alzheimer's," *Johns Hopkins Gazette* (March 17, 1997):www.jhu.edu/~gazette/ janmar97/mar1797/briefs.html.
10. Page, *Healthy Healing*, H422.
11. Source retrieved from the Internet October 22, 2002: Kevin Lamb, "Men can lead longer, healthier lives," *The Salina Journal* (July 24, 2002): www.saljournal.com/stories/ 072402/lif_health2.html.
12. Source retrieved from the Internet October 22, 2002: Edward Giovannucci et al., "A Prospective Study of Tomato Products, Lycopene, and Prostate Cancer Risk," *Journal of the National Cancer Institute* 94 (March 6, 2002): 391–398; http://jncicancerspectrum.oupjournals.org.
13. Janet Maccaro, Ph.D., C.N.C., *Breaking the Grip of Dangerous Emotions* (Lake Mary, FL: Siloam Press, 2001), 39–40.
14. Ibid.
15. Ibid.
16. Page, *Healthy Healing*, A317.
17. Ibid.
18. More information and statistics can be found on the Wobenzym website: www.wobenzym.com.
19. R. Ruane and P. Griffiths, "Glucosamine therapy compared to Ibuprofen for joint pain," *Br J Community Nurs* 7 (March 2002): 148–152.
20. Page, *Healthy Healing*, 319.
21. Richard N. Firshein, D.O., *Reversing Asthma* (New York: Warner Books, 1998).
22. Page, *Healthy Healing*, B324.

23. Billie J. Sahley, *The Anxiety Epidemic* (San Antonio, TX: Pain and Stress Publications, 1997).

24. Kari Watson, "The Brain's Balancing Act," *Natural Health Magazine* (September/October 1998): 60–69.

25. Ibid.

26. Paul Barney, M.D., *Doctor's Guide to Natural Medicine* (Pleasant Grove, UT: Woodland Publishing, Inc., 1998), 172.

27. N. Pashby et al., "A Clinical Trial of Evening Primrose Oil in Nastalgia," *Bri. Jour. Surg.* 68 (1981): 801–824.

28. P. R. Band et al., "Treatment of Benign Breast Disease with Vitamin A," *Prev Medicine* 13 (September 1984): 549–554.

29. Page, *Healthy Healing*, 339.

30. Ibid.

31. Linda Cook et al., "Perineal Powder Exposure and the Risk of Ovarian Cancer," *American Journal of Epidemiology* 145 (March 1997): 459–465.

32. Page, *Healthy Healing*, C336.

33. Source retrieved from the Internet October 22, 2002: American Cancer Society Guidelines for the Early Detection of Cancer (February 14, 2001): www.cancer.org.

34. R. Mas et al., "Effects of policosanol in patients with type II hypercholesterolemia and additional coronary risk factors," *Clinical Pharmacology Ther.* 65 (1999): 439–447.

35. Barney, *Doctor's Guide to Natural Medicine*, 184.

36. Page, *Healthy Healing*, C356.

37. November 1998 double-blind, placebo-controlled study in *Journal of the American Medical Association*, quoted in 2002 catalog from the Pain and Stress Center, San Antonio, TX.

38. Source retrieved from the Internet October 22, 2002: St. John's Wort, wholehealthmd.com: www.wholehealth.com/refshelf.

39. Page, *Healthy Healing*, C360.

40. Ibid., B324.

41. Interview by author with Michael T. Maccaro, D.M.D., 2002.

42. Ibid.

43. Sahley, *The Anxiety Epidemic*, 65–66.

44. Maccaro, *Breaking the Grip of Dangerous Emotions*, 178–179.

45. J. Wright and J. Burton, "Oral Evening Primrose Oil improves eczema," *Lancet* 2 (1982): 1120.

46. National Diabetes Statistics: General Information and National Estimates on Diabetes in the United States, 2000, NIH Publication No. 02-3892 (March 2002).

47. Hans-Michael Dosch et al., "Lack of Immunity to Bovine Serum Albumin in Insulin-Dependent Diabetes Mellitus," *New England Journal of Medicine* 330 (June 2, 1994): 1616–1617.

48. Page, *Healthy Healing*, D371.

49. W. J. Elliott and L. H. Powell, "Diagonal earlobe creases and prognosis in patients with suspected coronary artery disease," *American Journal of Medicine* 100 (February 1996): 205–211.

50. Billie J. Sahley, Ph.D., C.N.C., *Malic Acid and Magnesium for Fibromyalgia and Chronic Pain* (San Antonio, TX: Pain and Stress Publications, 1999).

51. Page, *Healthy Healing*.

52. Page, *Healthy Healing*, 405.

53. Ibid., 407.

54. P. H. Langsjoen and A. M. Langsjoen, "Overview of the Use of COQ10 in Cardiovascular Disease," *Biofactors* 9 (1999): 273–284.

55. Source retrieved from the Internet October 22, 2002: Hepatitis B Factsheet, American Liver Foundation, www.liverfoundation.org.

56. Source retrieved from the Internet October 22, 2002: Hepatitis A Factsheet, American Liver Foundation, www.liverfoundation.org

57. Page, *Healthy Healing*, H428.

58. *American Journal of Clinical Nutrition* (1977): 613.
59. *Lancet* (1977): 834–836.
60. *American Journal of Clinical Nutrition* 50: 851–867.
61. L. R. Juneja et al., "L-theanine—a unique amino acid of green tea and its relaxation effect in humans," *Trends Food Sci Tech* 10: 199–204.
62. Page, *Healthy Healing*, L447.
63. Balch and Balch, *Prescription for Nutritional Healing*, 443.
64. Sherry Kahn, M.P.H., "What's Your PMS Type?", *GreatLife* (June 2002): 18.
65. M. Yakir, S. Kreitler, A. Brzezinski et al., "Effects of homeopathic treatment in women with premenstrual syndrome: A pilot study," *British Homeopathic Journal* 90 (2001): 148–153. Also, Kahn, "What's Your PMS Type?"
66. Page, *Healthy Healing*, 496.
67. Giller and Matthews, *Medical Makeover*, 236–252.
68. Ibid.
69. Reprinted by permission of the Midwest Center for Stress and Anxiety, 106 N. Church St., P. O. Box 205, Oak Harbor, OH 43499. Phone: 800-511-6896; fax: 419-898-0669.
70. Ibid.
71. Sahley, *The Anxiety Epidemic*, 20.
72. Ibid.
73. Sandra Blakeslee, "Complex and Hidden Brain in Gut Makes Stomachaches and Butterflies," *New York Times* (January 23, 1996): C1.
74. Leo Galland, M.D., *GreatLife* (October 1998): 36–37.
75. Page, *Healthy Healing*, 518–520.
76. *The Daytona Beach News Journal* Wire Services, August 25, 2002

PART 4: SELF-TESTS AND NATURAL BODY MAINTENANCE

1. T. H. Holmes and R. H. Rahe, "The social readjustment rating scale," *Journal of Psychosomatic Research* 2 (1967): 213–218.
2. Page, *Healthy Healing*.

APPENDIX C: STRESS BUSTERS FROM NATURE

1. Linde Klaus et al., "St. John's wort for depression—an overview and meta-analysis of randomised clinical trials," *British Medical Journal* 313 (3 August 1996): 253–258.
2. H. P. Volz and M. Kieser, "Kava-kava extract WS 1490 versus placebo in anxiety disorders—a randomized placebo-controlled study 25-week outpatient trial," *Pharmacopsychiatry* 1 (January 30, 1997): 1–5.
3. *Natural Health* (November/December 1998): 168–172.
4. Ray Sahelian, M.D., 5-HTP: *Nature's Serotonin Solution* (n. p.: Avery Publishing Group, 1998.)

APPENDIX F: CLA = WEIGHT LOSS

1. Source obtained from the Internet: CLA (Conjugated Linoleic Acid), retrieved from www.painstresscenter.com/mall/CLA.asp.

PRODUCT INFORMATION

M ost of the products listed in *Natural Health Remedies* can be purchased at any health food store in America. Here is a list of resources for particular products mentioned in this book.

Dr. Janet's Balanced by Nature Products, Inc.
Visit www.DrjanetPhd.com for more information.
Products: Glucosamine Cream, Woman's Balance Formula/ Progesterone Cream, Men's Balance Formula, Skin Cream, SkinTastic Body Wash, Safe Passage menopause formula and Tranquility stress-relieving formula.

Nature's Secret/Omni Nutraceuticals
5310 Beethoven St., Los Angeles, CA 90066
800-297-3273
Products: Nature's Secret Ultimate Cleanse, Nature's Secret Ultimate Oil

Wakunaga of America, Ltd.
23501 Madero, Mission Viejo, CA 92691-2764
800-421-2998 (orders and sales)
Products: Kyo-Green, Kyolic Garlic, Kyo-Dophilus

Pain and Stress Center Products
5282 Medical Dr., # 160, San Antonio, TX 78229-6023
800-669-2256 (orders and sales)
Products: L-Theanine, GABA 750, Anxiety Control Formula, Amino Acid Profile Test, Brain Link, Liquid Serotonin, Sleep Link* Ask for catalogue on all anxiety and depression related products.

Tom's of Maine
P. O. Box 710, Keenebunk, ME 04043
800-367-8667 (orders)
Product: Natural Toothpaste

Enzymedica Therapeutic Enzymes
1625 West Marion Ave.
Punta Gorda, FL 33950
888-918-1118
Products: Digest, Lypo, Purify, Repair

Carlson Laboratories, Inc.
15 College Dr., Arlington Heights, IL 60004-1985
800-323-4141 (orders)
Product: Carlson's ACES and Liquid Magnesium gel capsules

Natrol, Inc.
20731 Marilla St., Chatsworth, CA 91311
800-326-1520
Product: Ester C

Candida Wellness Center
4365 N. Bedford Dr., Provo, UT 84604
800-869-1613
www.candidayeast.com
Product: Biotic Silver

Rodan and Fields Proactiv
Proactivsolution.com
800-333-0153
Product: proactiv

NOW Foods
550 Mitchell Rd., Glendale Heights, IL 60139
800-999-8069
Products: Stevia Extract Powder, Stevia Extract Liquid

Nutri-West of Florida
Products available through health professionals only.
800-451-5620
Core Level Adrenal

References and
Suggested Reading

The following health books and authors have been instrumental in bringing outstanding information in regards to the dietary and lifestyle links to disease and mental unrest. Their work has always been an inspiration to me and has influenced my work in a profound way. For further information on any of the given topics in my book, I suggest that you read the following books:

Balch, James F., M.D. and Phyllis A Balch, C.N.C. *Prescription for Nutritional Healing,* 2nd Edition. New York: Avery Publishing, 1997.

Barney, Paul, M.D. *Doctor's Guide to Natural Medicine.* Pleasant Grove, UT: Woodland Publishing, Inc., 1998.

Fuch, Nan Kathryn. *Woman's Health Letter.* Atlanta, GA: Sound View Publications, Inc. Call 800-728-2288 to subscribe or for more information.

Kaufman, Doug. *The Fungus Link.* Mediatrition, 2001.

Kreutle, Sylvia, M.S. *Nutritional Symptomatology Questionnaire.* Fort Collins, CO: HealthQuest, Inc. Sylvia Kreutle received a combined master's degree from Colorado State University in human nutrition and exercise physiology. She is the founder of HealthQuest, Inc., a company that provides health education materials and seminars for licensed professionals across the country. She has considerable background knowledge in clinical nutrition and over ten years of practical experience as an instructor, consultant and researcher.

Lang, J. Stephen. *Biblical Quotations for All Occasions.* N.p: Prima Publishing, 1999.

Maccaro, Janet, Ph.D., C.N.C. *90-Day Immune System Makeover.* Lake Mary, FL: Siloam Press, 2000.

———. *Breaking the Grip of Dangerous Emotions.* Lake Mary, FL: Siloam Press, 2001.

Page, Linda. *Healthy Healing,* 11th edition. N.p.: Traditional Wisdom, Inc., 2000.

Sahley, Billie J. *The Anxiety Epidemic.* San Antonio, TX: Pain and Stress Publications, 1997. Call 800-669-2256 to order or to obtain more information.

The Book of 1,000 Home Health Remedies. Peachtree City, GA: Frank W. Cawood and Associates, 1993.

The PDR Family Guide, Encyclopedia of Medical Care. New York: Three Rivers Press, 1997.

The World's Greatest Treasury of Health Secrets. N.p.: Bottomline Publications/Boardroom, Inc., 2002.

Walker, Norman W. *Fresh Vegetable and Fruit Juices.* Prescott, AZ: Norwalk Press, 1970. Call 800-205-2350 to order books.

For Further Help

National Alzheimer's Association
919 North Michigan Ave. #1100
Chicago, IL 60611
800-272-3900

National Women's Health Info Center
165 W. 46th St., Suite 1108
New York, New York 10036
212-575-6200
Website: www.4women.gov/nwhic/
    references/mdreferrals/aaba.htm

American Heart Association
National Center
7272 Greenville Ave.
Dallas, TX 75231
800-242-8721

Anxiety Disorders Association
    of America
8730 Georgia Ave., Ste. 600
Silver Spring, MD 20910
240-485-1001
Website: www.adaa.org

The CFIDS Association of America, Inc.
(Chronic Fatigue and Immune
    Dysfunction Syndrome Foundation)
P. O. Box 220398
Charlotte, NC 28222-0398
800-442-3437
Website: www.cfids.org

National Kidney Foundation
30 East 33rd St., Suite 1100
New York, NY 10016
800-622-9010
Website: www.kidney.org

American Cancer Society
1599 Clifton Rd.
Atlanta, GA 30329
24-hour HOTLINE: 800-ACS-2345

Lupus Foundation of America
1300 Piccard Drive, Suite 200
Rockville, MD 20850-4303
800-558-0121 (for information)
301-670-9292 (to talk to a nurse)
Website: www.lupus.org

Arthritis Foundation
P. O. Box 7669
Atlanta, GA 30357-0669
800-283-7800
Website: www.arthritis.org

The Food Allergy and
    Anaphylaxis Network
10400 Eaton Place, Suite 107
Fairfax, VA 22030-2208
800-929-4040
Website: www.foodallergy.org

Crohn's and Colitis Foundation
    of America
386 Park Avenue South, 17th Floor
New York, NY 10016
800-932-2423
Website: www.ccfa.org
E-mail: info@ccfa.org

A WOMAN'S BODY BALANCED BY NATURE

A PERSONAL HEALTH-BUILDING APPOINTMENT WITH DR. JANET

Audiotape Series (includes personal profile)

Wouldn't you love to sit down with Dr. Janet and receive a complete personal evaluation? This tape series is like having your own personal appointment with Dr. Janet as she walks you through a step-by-step personal health screening. As you listen to the tapes, you will complete a personal profile that will be your guide to understanding your body and its specific needs. You will have a plan for balancing and maintaining a healthy mind, body and spirit naturally. This series gives you:

- ❦ What foods to eat and avoid for your body type
- ❦ The latest information on preventing breast cancer and heart disease
- ❦ Keys to hormonal and body balancing
- ❦ Beneficial food list and eating combinations

Balanced by Nature Products Package (includes audiotape series, personal evaluation and Dr. Janet's Woman's Balance Formula cream)

This package combines the tape series with Dr. Janet's Balance Formula cream, which contains progesterone cream to give you everything you need—including step-by-step instructions to get you back on tract to a balanced, naturally healthy life—physically and emotionally. *Don't miss your appointment with Dr. Janet!*

To order, visit www.DrJanetPhD.com.

Don't stop now!

You're on the road to good health...
keep moving forward!

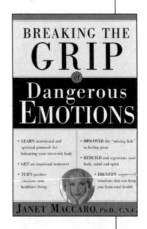
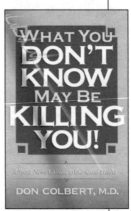
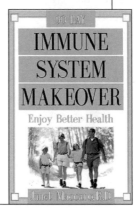
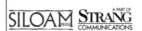